Anemia
From Molecule to Medicine

Isaias Raw, M.D.
Professor of Biochemistry and Nutrition
City College Center for Biomedical Education
City University of New York

The Foundations of Medical Science Series

Little, Brown and Company, Boston

Preface

By tradition, all over the world, the medical student has to work through a sequence of disciplines that begins with the basic biomedical sciences, continues with the clinical sciences, and is complete by hospital internship.

The disciplines still bear the same names, and in many traditional schools the same slice of teaching time, as when they were established more than half a century ago, when most of the knowledge available today was nonexistent. Updating has consisted mainly in the addition of new disciplines and has resulted in a continuous atomization of knowledge. This atomization leads frequently to overlaps and unplanned repetition of subject matter but fails to integrate the different disciplines.

This book is an example of how one disease entity can serve as a focus around which the student can pull together several disciplines and see how they support each other. It is the first of a projected series that is being prepared to foster an experiment in medical education. It is part of an attempt to challenge medical education to move away from its traditional structure by merging the basic and clinical sciences and rebuilding them into single learning units (to be used for learning, not lecturing) on a foundation of the motivation toward clinical medicine and of interest in all fields affecting it that every student has when he enters medical school.

The speed with which knowledge is now accumulating is such that we cannot expect to teach, nor the student to recall, everything in the field of medicine. Still more information will amass while the student is passing through medical school, and the accretion will continue forever. This volume is an attempt to create a model for a new way of structuring medical knowledge so that the student, and finally the practicing physician, will be better able to apply future discoveries.

How may a discovery in chemistry affect the choice of drugs he prescribes in clinical practice? What effect does a new fact of genetics have on his counseling of patients? When might the hierarchy of disease, from fatal to less serious, change because of a new understanding of and possibility of manipulating molecular structure? The kind of approach taken in this book can be used in any biomedical problem and can stand as a foundation for continuing medical education.

Anemia was selected as the focal topic for several reasons. It is one of the most common diseases and is therefore a real and relevant problem. Hemoglobin is the best-known biological macromolecule, and its complex functions can be understood in molecular terms. The covalent structure of this large polymer determines its tridimensional structure, and this determination thereby illustrates the economy with which information is stored in biological systems. Stored information is transmitted from parents to descendants and translated into the production of new molecules. Defects in this information, and other abnormalities, lead to a group of diseases known as anemias, which can be understood in their physiopathological details. Statistical knowledge of how often and by what family members the abnormalities are transmitted can be used in genetic counseling. Therefore it is possible, in studying anemia, to integrate a course of study running from molecules, through the organism, to the individual in whom the disease is diagnosed, and on to society itself. The student is shown the huge advances of modern biomedical research, the limits on its present application, and its potential for the future.

It is hoped that social and preventive medicine will be a part of this integration of disciplines, changing the attitudes of new doctors toward the social responsibilities of medical care.

There are a number of other diseases for which such conceptual structures could be built, interrelating physiopathological mechanisms, problems of prevention or cure, and sociomedical problems.

Until now this project has been a solitary effort, limited to the capabilities of one author, but steps have been taken to attract the cooperation of workers in several countries. I hope it will be possible to obtain contributions from specialists in basic, clinical, behavioral, and social medicine for the development of future models in the series, dealing with malnutrition, diabetes, diarrhea, trauma, and many other topics.

I. R.

New York City

Acknowledgments

This volume is the natural outcome of my experience in introducing innovations in medical and science education in Brazil. The distillation of that experience was made possible only by a combination of circumstances in Cambridge, Massachusetts. I am indebted to Prof. J. Zacharias, pioneer in so many areas of education, who provided me with the opportunity and with encouragement. The book itself was made possible by a grant from the Ford Foundation, which has supported many of my ventures in the past and helped me build my professional life in this country.

I thank the Departments of Biology and Nutrition of M. I. T. for receiving me as visiting professor and the students — some took the course on which this book is based — with whom I shared many hours of active interchange. I also acknowledge the help of the Pan-American Health Organization, which made possible an interchange with several leading Latin American groups.

The work on this book was completed while I was Visiting Professor of Health and Nutrition Education at the Harvard School of Public Health, and I am grateful to Fredrick Stare, Head of the Department of Nutrition, and Howard Hiatt, Dean, for their support.

Finally I would like to dedicate this volume to Zenaide and Silvia, my wife and daughter, who share and suffer for the years of efforts to innovate education in my country.

Introduction

If your watch is not working, you can find a skilled person to open it, inspect its parts, and replace the defective ones. If your television set does not operate, the repairman will try by a somewhat more indirect method to find what is wrong. He cannot open and inspect all the hundreds of components, but if he sees that there is no audio and the image is good, he will check only the parts of the circuit that deal with the sound.

Man is a similar system, even more complex. When a patient comes to you he will expect you to be able to find out what is wrong. He does not expect you routinely to open his body, however, and if you were to do so, often there would be nothing visibly wrong.

Let us imagine as a model an opaque plastic bag, presented as a problem. One could start by asking a few questions like "Is it a common object, or something special?" These questions are asked to limit the possibilities, and they resemble those commonly raised by a doctor who asks, "When did the present illness start? How was your health before?" This is the *clinical history,* which provides the doctor with a record of complaints, antecedent history, and family history, and enables him to uncover symptoms of which the patient himself is not fully aware.

Returning to the model, the next step would be to examine the bag, which would provide quite a large amount of information: The bag seems heavy, and by moving it you can tell that it is full of liquid. You can percuss the bag, that is, place the middle finger of your left hand on the bag and strike that finger with a sharp blow with the right hand. By the sound you may be able to tell whether the bag contains air as well as liquid. You may shake the bag and maybe you will be able to hear sounds if any objects are inside. This procedure is analogous to the *physical examination* that a practicing physician conducts.

You also may ask for an x-ray, and in this case you will see the outlines of objects inside, so you are thus able to describe their shape and number. Finally you can puncture the bag with a syringe and remove a small amount of liquid. If it looks like rusty water, and you can confirm the appearance by chemical analysis, it is likely that the objects in the bag are made of iron. This step compares with the *laboratory examination* performed in the clinical laboratory.

During the study of the module in this book, your problem is indeed realistic: man with anemia, one of the most common diseases. While you study these units, you may be able to obtain access to a clinic to study some medical cases. You will find out that you can make a diagnosis of anemia and understand its nature.

In the appendixes you will find more information about some important techniques.

Contents

Preface v
Acknowledgments vii
Introduction ix

1 INVESTIGATING THE RED CELL   **1**

Study Guide 1   Laboratory Investigation: Red Cells 2
Structure of the Red Cell Membrane 5   The Donnan
Equilibrium 9   Mediated Transport 11   Prevention of
Hemolysis 13   Laboratory Investigation: Hemoglobin
Content of Red Cells 13   Self-Evaluation 15   Further
Readings 16

2 FROM MOLECULES TO FUNCTION   **17**

Study Guide 17   Laboratory Investigation: Structure of
Hemoglobin 18   Molecular Structure of Hemoglobin 22
Laboratory Investigation: Properties of Hemoglobin 38
Physiological Role of Hemoglobin 39   Self-Evaluation 43
Further Readings 44

3 FROM MOLECULES TO DISEASE   **47**

Study Guide 47   Laboratory Investigation: Experimental
Anemia 48   Anemia 48   Laboratory Investigation:
Diagnosis of Anemias 52   Globin Defects 53
Metabolic Defects 55   Membrane Defects 55
Laboratory Investigation: Blood and Bone Smears 56
Self-Evaluation 57 Alterations in Osmotic and Mechanical
Fragility Related to In Vivo Erythrocyte Aging and Splenic

Sequestration in Hereditary Spherocytosis (Robert C. Griggs, Russel Weisman, Jr., and John W. Harris) *59 Further Readings 75*

4 FROM MOLECULES TO GENETICS 77

Study Guide 77 Mendel's Laws 77 Laboratory Investigation: Hereditary Traits 78 Dominance 79 Ratios 81 Laboratory Investigation: Human Genetics 83 Genetic Counseling 84 Genetic Control of Hemoglobin Synthesis 85 Sex-Linked Traits 97 Group Discussion: Genetic Counseling 100 Self-Evaluation 100 The Separation of Glucose-6-Phosphate-Dehydrogenase-Deficient Erythrocytes from the Blood of Heterozygotes for Glucose-6-Phosphate-Dehydrogenase Deficiency (Ernest Beutler and Maryellen C. Baluda) *102 Further Readings 111*

5 FROM MOLECULES TO INFORMATION 113

Study Guide 113 Genetic Information 114 Mitosis 114 Meiosis 115 Crossing-Over 117 Chemical Composition of Genetic Information 118 The Watson and Crick Model 124 Molecular Structure of Nucleic Acids: A Structure for Deoxyribose Nucleic Acid (J. D. Watson and F. H. C. Crick) *125* Genetical Implications of the Structure of Deoxyribonucleic Acid (J. D. Watson and F. H. C. Crick) *128 Laboratory Investigation: Properties of DNA 135 DNA Structure and Replication 140 Laboratory Investigation: Chromosomes 141 DNA and Chromosomes 144 Transcribing the Message 152* The Enzymatic Incorporation of Ribonucleotides into RNA and the Role of DNA (Tables) (Jerard Hurwitz, J. J. Furth, Monika Anders, P. J. Ortiz, and J. T. August) *154 Hybridization 160 The Role of Soluble RNA 161 Ribosomes and Protein Synthesis 165 Ribosomes and the Nucleolus 173 Breaking the Code 176 Erythropoietin and Hemoglobin Synthesis 180 Self-Evaluation 182 Hemoglobin Synthesis: A Round Table Discussion 183 Further Readings 184 Annual Reviews 184*

6 MOLECULES TO POPULATION   **185**

*Study Guide 185   Hardy-Weinberg Law 186
Consanguinity 189   Selection 192   Genetic Load 195
Eugeny 196   Self-Evaluation 197*   Protection Afforded
by Sickle-Cell Trait against Subtertian Malarial Infection (A. C.
Allison) *198   Further Readings 207*

APPENDIXES   **209**
  I Medical History Questionnaire   **211**
 II Electrophoresis   **219**
III Centrifugation   **223**
IV Chromatography   **227**
 V PH, Titration, Buffers   **231**
VI Probability and Statistics   **237**

*Answers to Self-Evaluation Tests 247
Index 251*

Anemia
From Molecule to Medicine

1   Investigating the Red Cell

STUDY GUIDE

This unit describes the red cell, its chemical constituents, and its equilibrium with the medium surrounding it. After reading the text and conducting the experiments you should be able to do the following:

1. Describe the structure of the red cell membrane.

2. Explain how molecules and ions are transported through this membrane and what physicochemical principles are involved in the process.

3. Explain the concept of transport mediated by a permease, and give evidence to back it.

4. State the precautions necessary to preserve red cells from hemolysis, and be able to explain how to separate and preserve red cells in vitro.

5. State the precautions that should be taken to avoid hemolysis when solutions are to be injected into the bloodstream.

6. Obtain a blood sample, and prepare and stain smears.

7. Use the microscope to count cells, recognize their shapes, and measure them.

8. Do a hematocrit determination.

9. Use a chromatography to purify a protein.

LABORATORY INVESTIGATION: RED CELLS

1. Examine your own blood to find out about the red cell: What is its shape? Does it have a nucleus like other cells? How many red cells are there in 1 ml of blood? What volume of blood is due to the red cells? What is the average volume of one red cell? What is the average diameter of a red cell? Are they all the same size? Can you substantiate your answer with a statistical treatment? Are the values you found for red cells normal?

2. Investigate what happens when you suspend red cells in (a) water, (b) different concentrations of sodium chloride (0.6, 0.9, 1.2, and 1.5 g/liter), and (c) 0.25M urea. Find out if you can preserve red cells by freezing.

Study the procedures described below. You may want to refer to some of the general laboratory methods described in the appendices. Plan the experiments in advance, discuss them with the instructor, and after performing them prepare a short report with the results obtained and your conclusions.

Procedure for Obtaining Blood

For the first part of the laboratory investigation a small blood sample is required, which can be obtained from your own fingertip. In a small watch glass, prepare 0.03 ml of anticoagulant (1.2 g ammonium oxalate and 0.8 g potassium oxalate in 100 ml of water) and let dry. Clean the tip of your finger with alcohol and let dry. Puncture with a sterile lancet; wipe away the first drop of blood. Collect a few drops of blood in the watch glass, swirling to mix with the anticoagulant. If you need to dilute the blood sample, use 0.9% sodium chloride.

Measuring the Volume of Red Cells with the Hematocrit

Take a special capillary tube with a plastic cap and fill it with blood. (If you are taking blood directly from the fingertip, use a capillary tube that is coated with heparin, an anticoagulant.) Cap the tube and put it to spin in a centrifuge. There are special heads to hold capillary tubes, but these are not necessary; you may use a common centrifuge with some cotton inside the tube holder. Spin for 2 minutes at about 3,000 rpm. Measure the total height of the blood and the height of the red cells. The relative volume of red cells to whole blood can then be obtained.

Counting Red Cells

Use a blood cell counting kit that has a special micropipette with marks at 0.05 and at 1.01 ml. With the pipette, draw up enough blood to reach the 0.05 mark. Wipe the tip. Now, while rotating the pipette on its longitudinal axis, draw up enough Hayden solution (0.5 g mercuric chloride and 5 g sodium chloride in 200 ml water) to reach the 1.01 mark. Hold the pipette with one hand, so that your fingers close both ends, and mix by carefully turning the pipette upside down and back several times. This dilutes the blood 1:200.

Put the special cover slide on the counting chamber. Fill the ruled area with the diluted blood, avoiding bubbles. Using the microscope, count the red cells in the five areas designated in the diagram (Fig. 1-1). Since the chamber is

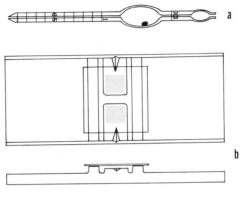

a

b

Fig. 1-1. Hemocytometer. (a) diluting pipette; (b) chamber; (c) ruled grid showing counting areas.

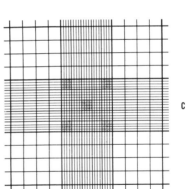

c

0.1 mm deep, and the surface area counted is 0.2 mm^2, the red cells counted fill 0.02 mm^3. Since the blood was diluted 1:200 (0.005), the cell count is $0.02 \times 0.005 = 0.0001$ mm^3. This number should be multiplied by 10^4 to find red cells per cubic millimeter.

Measuring with the Microscope

Some microscopes come equipped with a disc with an engraved ruled scale. The manufacturer's instructions give the value of each division of this scale, for different objectives.

If you have just a ruled scale disc with no specified values, insert it inside the ocular. To find out how much each division represents, for a selected objective, focus on the red cell counting chamber. The side of the small square measures 0.05 mm.

Staining Red Cells for Examination

Mix a drop of blood with a drop of methylene blue solution (0.5 g new methylene blue, 1.4 g potassium oxalate, 0.8 g sodium chloride, and water up to 100 ml). After ten minutes spread it on a slide by means of a cover slide, as shown in Figure 1-2. Let it dry, and examine under high power.

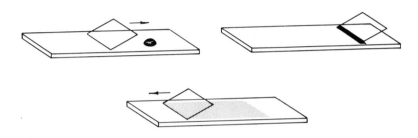

Fig. 1-2. Preparing a blood smear.

Red Cell Preparation

For the second part of the laboratory investigation, you will need more blood. Learn the proper procedure for taking blood from a person's vein, and obtain a 5 ml blood sample. Using a dry sterile syringe, transfer the sample to a tube in which 0.5 ml of anticoagulant has been dried. Mix carefully. Dilute the blood with about 20 ml 0.9% sodium chloride, and centrifuge. The red cells will collect at the bottom of the tube. Discard the supernatant. Resuspend in 0.9% sodium chloride, centrifuge, and discard the supernatant. Resuspend the red cells in 10 ml of 0.9% sodium chloride. Take 0.5 ml of the cell suspension, centrifuge, and resuspend using the various suspensions given in item 2.

Normal Values

Table 1-1. Normal Values for the Red Blood Cell

Subject	Hematocrit (%)	Cells (10^6/mm^3)	Volume[a] (μ^3)	Diameter (μ)
At birth	56±10	4.8−7.1	77	8.2
First year	35± 5	4.0−5.5	106	
Males	47± 7	4.6−6.2	87	7−7.5
Females	42± 5	4.2−5.4	87	7−7.5

[a]The volume (mean corpuscular volume or MCV) is calculated by dividing (hematocrit × 10) by the millions of red cells/mm^3.

STRUCTURE OF THE RED CELL MEMBRANE

Permeability of Red Cells

Experiments with plant and animal cells and their membranes led to the discovery of *osmosis*. There are some membranes that will allow the passage of water molecules but not of certain chemicals dissolved in the water. If two solutions of different concentrations are separated by such a membrane, water will pass from the less concentrated to the more concentrated solution until the two concentrations become equal. If the more concentrated solution is connected to a manometer (Fig. 1-3), the migration of water will make the

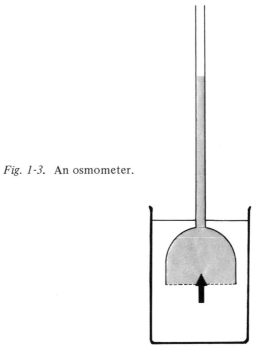

Fig. 1-3. An osmometer.

manometer rise, showing an increase in pressure. The flow of water will continue until the water pressure balances the tendency of water to diffuse in. Measuring the amount of increase in water pressure is one method of measuring the osmotic pressure.

Van't Hoff made a fundamental contribution when he discovered that the osmotic pressure was dependent on concentration, as represented by the *number* of particles (such as molecules or ions) in a volume of solution, and not on their size or weight. The osmotic pressure of dilute solutions follows the ideal gas law

$$\pi = \frac{nRT}{V}$$

where π is the osmotic pressure, n the number of moles in the volume V, R the gas constant, and T the absolute temperature.

Like osmotic pressure, the freezing point depression and the boiling point elevation of solutions (as compared to pure solvents) are *colligative* properties; that is, they depend on the number but not the nature of the particles dissolved. The freezing point is frequently used to find the total concentration of molecules and ions in blood plasma, since it is more quickly and easily measured than osmotic pressure.

Isotonic Concentration

By suspending red cells in different concentrations of sucrose and observing the size and shape of the cells, one can determine the *isotonic* concentration of sucrose (the concentration having the same osmotic pressure as the red cell). It is found to be around 0.3*M*. For sodium chloride it is around 0.15*M*, because the NaCl molecules are entirely dissociated into two ions.

Hemolysis

In dilute solutions, water will migrate into the red cells by osmosis until the membrane bursts, releasing hemoglobin and the other contents of the cell. This is called *hemolysis*. In hypertonic glycerin (a solution that has higher osmotic pressure than the cytoplasm of red cells) red cells first shrink, then go back to their original size, continue to enlarge, and finally hemolyze. The explanation for this is simple: at first water migrates out of the cell, but glycerin penetrates slowly into the cell until it reaches the same concentration inside as it has outside, at which point the red cell is hypertonic in relation to the medium, and hemolyzes. Urea, on the other hand, penetrates cells rapidly and causes them to hemolyze quickly.

These experiments show the existence of a membrane that must have pores which allow water, glycerin, and urea to pass through. We also see that larger molecules such as sucrose or hemoglobin do not diffuse through the membrane. At the end of the last century, Overton discovered that the permeability of the red cell membrane to a number of substances is inversely proportional to their molecular diameter. This, of course, is what one expects if one starts from the idea of migration of molecules through the pores of the membrane. Overton studied over 500 substances and found a large number whose permeability was related not to their size but to their solubility in lipids. He postulated that these chemicals dissolve in the membrane and from there pass to the interior of the cell.

Lipoprotein Membrane

In 1925 Gortner and Grendal hemolyzed red cells and recovered the membranes by centrifugation. (Such recovered membranes are called *ghosts*.) On analyzing the membranes, they found lipids of a quantity sufficient to cover twice the surface of the red cells. Hence, they proposed the cell membrane structure to be a double layer of lipid molecules that oriented the groups soluble in water on the outside of either the cell or the cytoplasm, while the groups that were insoluble existed in the interior of the membrane. Years later it was found that the lipids of the red cell membrane are phospholipids that have at one end water-soluble (*polar*) groups and at the other water-insoluble (*non-polar*) groups, as Gortner postulated (Fig. 1-4).

Measurements of some of the properties of the membrane, such as electric capacitance and surface tension, did not agree with the idea of a lipid membrane. It was found that in the ghost there is a considerable amount of protein, twice as much by weight as lipid. The protein molecules are much larger than the lipid, however, so that there is a protein molecule for seventy phospholipid molecules. In 1935 Danielli and Dawson proposed that the membrane was a sandwich with protein layers outside and a double layer of phospholipids inside (Fig. 1-5). In 1959 Robertson improved the techniques of preparing materials for examination under the electron microscope, and obtained a picture clearly showing three layers of membrane with a total thickness of 7.5 nm. This agrees with the Danielli-Dawson model that has been accepted for many years.

Recently it was shown that it is possible to digest the membrane with an enzyme, phospholipase C. Although the molecule of the enzyme is quite large, it can reach and remove the phosphate groups of the phospholipids that are not masked by the proteins.

A more refined technique of examining fine structures under the electron microscope was developed recently: The material is rapidly frozen, placed at $-100°C$ under vacuum, and fractured by a sharp knife. The two outer layers of the red cell separate, and it is possible to see small particles of about 7.5 nm,

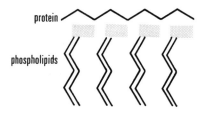

Fig. 1-4. Phospholipid molecule. Shaded area represents the polar end of the molecule.

protein

phospholipids

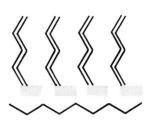

Fig. 1-5. Danielli-Dawson model for membrane structure.

which might represent little protein globules inserted in the double phospholipid layer. This model, proposed by Braton and Singer, can be represented as shown in Figure 1-6.

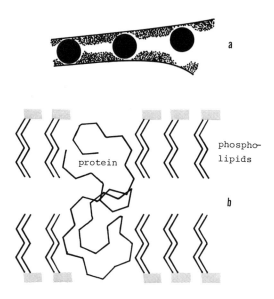

Fig. 1-6. Mosaic model for membrane structure, showing protein globules and lipids. (a) diagram of structure as seen by electron microscope after freezing and fracturing; (b) proposed molecular structure.

THE DONNAN EQUILIBRIUM

It is known that cells contain much more potassium and less sodium than the medium which surrounds them (Table 1-2). To explain this, one may use a model developed by Donnan in 1911 for a porous membrane separating two

Table 1-2. Concentration in Red Cells and Plasma.

Ions	(μMol/1)	
	Red Cells	Plasma
Na^+	19	140
K^+	136	41
Cl^-	72	115

solutions. Both solutions contain ions that can pass through the pores, but one contains a large molecule, like a protein, which cannot pass. Imagine that the protein under the conditions of this experiment behaves as an anion (p^-). Cl^- and Na^+ are also present. Starting with the same concentrations of sodium and protein on one side and sodium and chloride on the other. (Fig. 1-7), one

$Na^+ = 1.00$	$Na^+ = 1.00$
$Cl^- = 0.00$	$Cl^- = 1.00$
$Pr^- = 1.00$	

$Na^+ = 1.33$	$Na^+ = 0.67$
$Cl^- = 0.33$	$Cl^- = 0.67$
$Pr^- = 1.00$	

Fig. 1-7. Donnan equilibrium. Left, initial; right, final.

sees, as would be expected, that the chloride ions have a tendency to migrate to the inside, reaching equal concentrations on both sides. This leads to an electric imbalance, unless sodium also migrates. Even though sodium has the same concentration on both sides, migration will occur until the product of the diffusible ions on each side is equal (subscript $_i$ = inside and subscript $_o$ = outside)

$$(Na^+)_i \, (Cl^-)_i = (Na^+)_o \, (Cl^-)_o$$

and both sides are electrically neutral, meaning that the charge of the cations balances the charge of the anions. If we call the amount of chloride that migrates x, we have

$$(1 + x)(x) = (1 - x)(1 - x)$$

and then solving for x, we obtain the value 0.33.

In this equilibrium (called the *Donnan equilibrium*) one would expect there to be an osmotic imbalance resulting in water migration. Also, as the concentrations of sodium inside and outside are different, inserting one electrode inside and another outside should show an electric potential. This potential can indeed be measured by microelectrodes in living cells.

Calculations show that the Donnan equilibrium does not explain the high concentration of K^+ and low concentration of Na^+ in the red cells. To explain these abnormal concentrations it has been postulated that the red cell membrane is permeable to anions but not to cations.

In venous blood, carbon dioxide received from the tissues enters the red cell by being converted into bicarbonate ions. As one expects, these ions migrate to the plasma. Sodium or potassium cannot migrate outward to keep the electric balance. Instead, chloride migrates from the plasma exactly as calculated by the Donnan equilibrium (Fig. 1-8). The reverse occurs in the blood when it reaches the lung.

Fig. 1-8. Chloride shift.

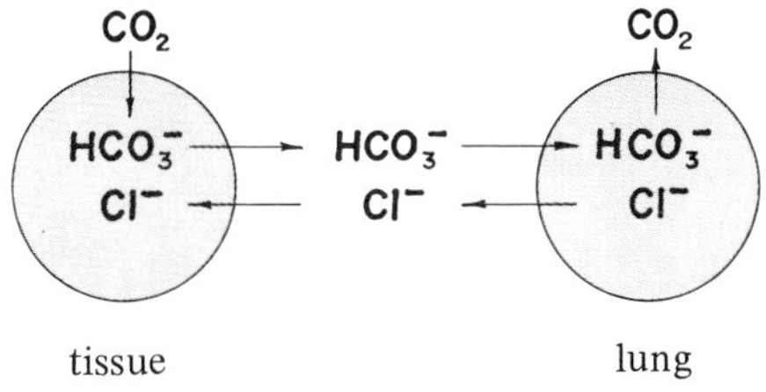

tissue   lung

During the early 1940s, when it became possible to produce radioactive potassium and sodium, it was found that those cations do pass rapidly through the membrane of the living red cell. If the red cell metabolism is blocked by cooling or by inhibitors of glucose metabolism, potassium leaks out and sodium comes in. This indicates that there is an active mechanism for red cell permeability, which, using energy generated by cell metabolism, continuously pumps out the sodium in exchange for the potassium.

MEDIATED TRANSPORT

Measurement of the rate of penetration of glucose into the red cell shows that the rate increases as the external concentration of glucose increases, until it reaches a maximum. Contrary to what one would expect from a simple porous membrane, further increasing the concentration of glucose does not increase the rate of permeability. Another interesting observation is that, although many sugars penetrate the red cells, others do not. D-Xylose penetrates, whereas the isomer L-xylose, the same size, does not. When two sugars that penetrate are mixed, the rate of permeability for each one is smaller than when each is alone. Furthermore, phloridzin, a chemical found in apple tree roots, inhibits the uptake of sugars.

These observations can be explained if one assumes the presence of a carrier (called a *permease*). This carrier should be specific, combining with glucose and some, but not all, other sugars at the outer surface of the cell membrane.

After so combining, the permease moves inside the membrane, or turns around, releasing the sugar within the cell's interior (Fig. 1-9). This continues until the concentration on both sides of the membrane is the same.

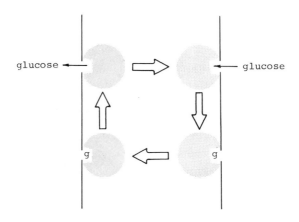

Fig. 1-9. Glucose transport mediated by permease.

Increasing the sugar concentration outside the cell should increase the chance that the sugar will combine with the permease. Above a certain concentration, when all the permease is already operating at full capacity, the rate of penetration reaches a maximum. Therefore the capacity of the permease to transfer the molecule to the inside is the limiting factor, not the concentration outside. If two sugars are mixed, each one tries to combine with the permease, and, as should be expected, the permeability of both is slowed down. The effect produced by phloridzin is explained by the fact that it combines with the permease, blocking its function.

If a red cell is placed in a medium with a sugar like 3-0-methyl-glucose until the concentration inside is the same as outside, and then glucose is added, as the glucose is transferred into the cell, the methyl-glucose is transferred to the outside even though it has already achieved a balanced concentration. What happens is that as the permease carries glucose from the outside, where it is concentrated, to the inside, methyl-glucose is carried out as a by-product. This common phenomenon in cell permeability is called *exchange diffusion.*

Red cells have other permeases. A specific one for glycerin exists which is blocked by trace amounts of copper. The amount of the various permeases is so small that it is difficult to isolate them, but some progress along this line has been made with bacterial cells.

PREVENTION OF HEMOLYSIS

Red cells cannot be preserved by freezing, since they hemolyze on thawing. It was once thought that the cause of this was formation of ice crystals that damaged the membrane. It was suggested that glycerin be used to prevent the formation of large ice crystals, and it was found that in $3M$ glycerin one can freeze red cells without hemolysis. This method is of value for preserving red cells and other tissues used for transplantation, but the initial rationale has been shown to be wrong. When red cells are kept in salt solutions, and the solution begins to freeze, ice crystals form. The remainder of the solution becomes hypertonic (with a higher osmotic pressure in relation to the red cell cytoplasm). Salts move into the red cells. On thawing, the outside becomes hypotonic, and water rushes into the cells, hemolyzing them. As glycerin is transported by a permease, its movement in and out of the cell prevents large osmotic differences in the thawing process.

LABORATORY INVESTIGATION: HEMOGLOBIN CONTENT OF RED CELLS

The purpose of this investigation is to measure the hemoglobin content per red cell and find out what proportion it represents of the red cell in relation to the total dry matter present.

Obtain purified hemoglobin by column chromatography. Use this purified sample to calibrate the photocolorimetric method for hemoglobin determination. Find the amount of hemoglobin present in the purified fraction by measuring the iron in it. Hemoglobin contains 0.34 percent iron.

Drying

Water can be removed by heating at about 60 to $70°C$. With this method there is a risk of destroying some heat-labile compounds or leaving water behind. It is a good precaution to dry again until the sample approaches a constant weight, to show that all water was removed.

If possible use lyophilization, a process which involves a high vacuum at low temperatures. This dehydrates the sample by sublimation of water without damaging the labile compounds.

Purification of Hemoglobin

Sephadex G-25 should be left to stand overnight in 5 volumes of distilled water. The next day prepare a chromatographic column about 1 cm in diameter and 50 cm high. A burette can be used for this, with some glass wool at the bottom. Pour in the Sephadex suspension, allowing the water to run out without ever letting the column go dry. Hemolyze a 1 ml red cell suspension with water, and centrifuge at high speed to remove the ghosts. Introduce the solution into the column and wash down with water aliquots. Collect the hemoglobin fraction, discarding the beginning and the end. Hemoglobin is red, so you should be able to determine which parts to discard.

Determination of Hemoglobin

Mix 0.02 ml of blood with 5 ml of ammonium hydroxide (4 mg/liter). Shake well and read in a photocolorimeter at 540 nm or with a green filter. Use a hemoglobin standard (or a blood with known hemoglobin concentration) to calibrate the method.

Table 1-3. Normal Values for Hemoglobin

Subject	Hemoglobin (g/100 ml blood)	MCHC[a] (%)
At birth	18.0–27.0	33–38
First year	9.0–14.6	33–38
Adult males	14.0–18.0	33–38
Adult females	11.5–16.0	33–38

[a]Mean corpuscular hemoglobin concentration = 100 × hemoglobin in g/100 divided by hematocrit

Determination of Iron

Transfer 0.5 ml of blood to a 50 ml volumetric flask. Add, swirling constantly, 3 ml of concentrated sulfuric acid, and keep agitating the flask for a few minutes. Now add 3 ml of a saturated solution of sodium persulfate (made fresh every week and containing 7 g/100 ml), and keep agitating for a few minutes more. Dilute to about 25 ml with water. Then add 2 ml of 10% sodium tungstate. Dilute the solution to 50 ml with water, mix, and filter.

Prepare an iron standard by dissolving exactly 0.861 g of Fe $NH_4(SO_4)_2 \cdot$ 12 H_2O in some distilled water. Add 2 ml of concentrated sulfuric acid and dilute to 1 liter. The standard has 0.1 mg of iron per milliliter.

To 15 ml of filtrate add 1 ml of potassium persulfate and 3 ml of potassium thiocyanate solution (made by dissolving 29.2 g potassium thiocyanate in about 90 ml water, adding 4 ml acetone, and diluting to exactly 100 ml). Dilute to 20 ml. Prepare a blank by using water instead of the filtrate, and a standard by using 0.6 ml of the iron standard. Treat them as you did the filtrate. Read the solutions at 540 nm or with a green filter.

SELF-EVALUATION

1. The hematocrit determination provides
   a. the concentration of hemoglobin in the blood.
   b. the number of red cells per cubic millimeter.
   c. the fraction of the blood volume due to red cells.
   d. the diameter of red cells.

2. The concentration of sodium inside the red cells is explained by
   a. the fact that the red cell membrane is impermeable to ions.
   b. osmosis and Donnan equilibrium.
   c. the existence of pores in a phospholipid membrane.
   d. permeases and active transport coupled with cell metabolism.

3. A 0.155*M* sodium chloride solution is isotonic. A 0.155*M* glucose solution would be
   a. hypotonic.
   b. isotonic.
   c. hypertonic.

4. If red cells are in a slightly suspended hypertonic glycerin solution
   a. the cells will shrink.
   b. the cells will shrink and then hemolyze.
   c. the cells will hemolyze immediately.
   d. the cells will maintain their shape.

5. Chloride shift describes
   a. the replacement of chloride by oxygen.
   b. the replacement of chloride by potassium ions.
   c. the replacement of chloride by bicarbonate ions.
   d. the movement of chloride ions that accompany sodium ions.

6. A hematocrit of 35 and a count of 4,800,000 red cells per cubic millimeter in an adult male
   a. is normal.
   b. shows a low number of red cells.
   c. represents a normal value for red cells and a low total red cell volume.
   d. shows a low hematocrit and a low red cell count.

FURTHER READINGS

Christensen, H. H.   *Biological Transport.*   New York: Benjamin, 1962.

Dowben, R. M.   *General Physiology.*   New York: Harper & Row, 1969.

Frankel, S., Reitman, S., and Sonnenwirth, A. C.   *Gradwohl's Clinical Laboratory Methods and Diagnosis.*   St. Louis, Mo.:   Mosby, 1970.

Harris, J. W., and Kellermeyer, R. W.   *The Red Cell.*   Cambridge, Mass.:   Harvard University Press, 1970.

Jameilson, G. A., and Greenwalt, T. J. (Eds.)   *Red Cell Membrane: Structure and Function.*   Philadelphia: Lippincott, 1969.

Rothfield, L. I.   *Structure and Function of Biological Membranes.*   New York: Academic, 1972.

Stein, W. D.   *The Movement of Molecules Across Cell Membranes.*   New York: Academic, 1967.

Turner, A. R.   *Frozen Blood.*   New York: Gordon and Breach, 1970.

Wolstenholme, G. E. W., and O'Connor, M. (Eds.)   *The Frozen Cell.*   Ciba Symposia.   Edinburgh and London: Churchill and Livingstone, 1970.

2 From Molecules to Function

STUDY GUIDE

The structure and properties of hemoglobin are considered here with a view to arriving at an understanding of the general structure of protein, and the relationship of structure to function is explored to explain how hemoglobin performs its role. After reading this chapter and doing some of the experiments you should be able to do the following.

1. Write the general formula for all amino acids and the specific formula for a few, and explain the way they link by peptide bonds.

2. Understand that proteins are linear polymers of up to 20 different kinds of amino acids, linked by peptide bonds; that these amino acids occur and recur in a specific sequence for each protein; and that this sequence may differ in only a few places in different species.

3. Describe the properties of polar and nonpolar groups and their role in establishing the tridimensional structure of proteins, and understand how this tridimensional structure is a direct consequence of the primary structure.

4. Understand that disturbing this natural tridimensional structure can result in new configurations, resulting in loss of some of the molecule's physical and biological properties.

5. Understand that hemoglobin contains iron as Fe^{++}, which combines reversibly with oxygen, and describe the participation of the rest of the molecule including the interaction of the four chains, that results in the transport of oxygen from the lungs to the tissues.

6. Titrate an amino acid to determine its pK and the buffer effect.

7. Describe the role of hemoglobin as a buffer in the transport of carbon dioxide from the tissues to the lungs.

8. Perform amino acid chromatography, using the basic techniques for determination of the amino acid sequence in a protein.

LABORATORY INVESTIGATION: STRUCTURE OF HEMOGLOBIN

Prepare globin by removing the heme from hemoglobin through the acid-acetone treatment. For purposes of comparison, use a sample of a small peptide that contains two or three amino acids. Study the structure of the two samples to identify the amino acids present and the terminal amino acid of a free amino group (see Figure 2-1).

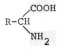

Fig. 2-1. Amino acid. Shaded area represents the free carboxyl and alpha amino groups.

Preparation of Globin

To prepare the globin, treat a sample of hemoglobin with an equal volume of cold acetone containing 2% hydrochloric acid. The protein will precipitate and can be separated by centrifugation. It should be washed with more cold acetone. This globin will be used as the protein in the methods that follow.

Protein Hydrolysis

Dissolve 10 mg of the protein precipitate (or 1 mg of the small peptide) in 2 ml of N hydrochloric acid in a test tube. Cap the tube with a glass marble and put it in an oven at $110°C$ for 6 to 24 hours. (In this procedure tryptophan and part of the serine are destroyed.)

Amino Acid Chromatography by Thin-Layer Chromatography (TLC)

Obtain a square, silica gel, thin-layer chromatograph sheet. Activate it by placing it in an oven at $100°C$ for half an hour, and let it cool. On the left corner, about 2 cm from the edges, place about 10 μl of the protein hydrolyzate.

Table 2-1. Silica Gel Thin-Layer Chromatography (numbers in body of table = $R_f \times 100$.

Amino Acids	Solvents[a]									
	For Amino Acids					For DNP—Amino Acids				
	1	2	3	4	5	6	7	8[b]	9[b]	10
Ala	37	22	29	39	47	54	60	32	59	....
Arg	02	06	19	10	04	....	....	....	....	43
Asn	....	14	....	....	....	....	....	....	....	....
Asp	33	17	06	09	55	13	09	06	07	....
$CySO_3H$	50	10	04	17	69	....	....	....	....	29
Gln	....	15	....	....	....	....	....	....	....	....
Glu	35	24	10	14	63	26	31	12	12	....
Gly	32	18	24	29	43	32	40	17	31	....
His	20	05	32	38	33	....	....	....	....	....
Lys-OH	....	....	04	....	44	....	....	....	....	....
Pro-OH	34	16	38	28	....	....	....	....	....	....
Ile	53	43	49	52	60	83	81	107	100	....
Leu	55	44	48	53	61	82	80	100	100	....
Lys	02	03	09	18	03	....	....	....	....	....
Met	51	35	49	51	59	70	69	43	72	....
Phe	58	43	55	54	63	75	74	44	81	....
Pro	26	14	50	37	35	65	38	58	78	....
Ser	35	18	20	27	48	11	11	09	07	....
Thr	37	20	26	37	50	17	15	12	09	....
Try	62	47	63	55	65	69	69	23	54	....
Tyr	57	41	47	42	65	....	....	....	....	....
Val	45	42	40	48	55	79	77	76	91	....
His-diDNP	....	....	....	....	....	11	08	05	12	....
Hys-imDNP	....	....	....	....	....	....	....	....	....	57
Lys-diDNP	....	....	....	....	....	56	60	12	66	....
Tyr-diDNP	....	....	....	....	....	58	60	17	57	....
Lys	....	....	....	....	....	....	....	....	....	44
DNP	....	....	....	....	....	100	83	22	148	....
$DNP-NH_2$	....	....	....	....	....	90	72	115	131	....

[a] 1. n-propanol—water 70:30
 2. N-butanol—glacial acetic acid—water 4:1:1
 3. phenol-water 75:25 (in weight)
 4. n-propanol—34% ammonium hydroxide 70:30
 5. 96% ethanol—water 70:30
 6. chloroform—benzil alcohol—glacial acetic acid 70:30:3
 7. chloroform—ter-amylalcohol—glacial acetic acid 70:30:3
 8. benzene—pyridine—glacial acetic acid 80:202
 9. chloroform—methanol—glacial acetic acid 95:5:1
10. for water-soluble DNP derivates with solvent 4
[b] R_f bases on R_f 100/or leucine.

The spot should not be more than 5 mm in diameter. Add part of the sample with a micropipette, and let it dry; repeat until all the sample has been added. (Chromatography will be performed twice, once with the globin sample and once with the peptide sample.)

Tape three edges of a glass plate with two layers adhesive tape. Place the TLC sheet on the glass plate, with the silica gel surface up, using a little vacuum grease to hold the plastic sheet to the glass. Cover with a second glass plate, securing with two bulldog clips. This plate should not touch the surface of the silica gel. Refer to Table 2-1 for a list of solvents and the respective R_f values for various amino acids (See also Appendix IV, Chromatography). Choose any two solvents for your chromatogram. Prepare a container with the first solvent. Put the lower edge of the glass plate into the solvent, and keep it there until the solvent has risen about 15 cm. Remove and open the plate, mark with a pencil the point to which the solvent has migrated, and let it dry.

Turn the TLC sheet 90 degrees, and add a standard containing a few known amino acids to the left corner. Replace the sheet between the glass plates, clamp, and place it in the second solvent (Fig. 2-2.). After the solvent has risen

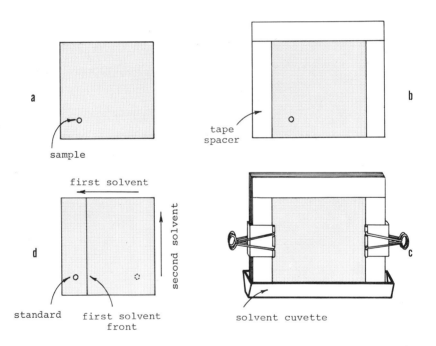

Fig. 2-2. Bidimensional thin-layer chromatography. (a) Apply the sample. (b) Place the thin layer sheet on the glass plate with the tape spacer. (c) Cover with the second glass plate, clamp, and insert in the cuvette with the solvent. (d) Remove the glass plate, mark the solvent front, dry, spot the standard, and reassemble for the second chromatography.

about 15 cm, remove the plate, mark the point of migration of the solvent, and let it dry. Spray with ninhydrin (made by dissolving 0.5 g of 1,2,3 triketohydrindene in 100 ml of ethanol and adding 4 ml of 2,4,6 collidine and 3 ml glacial acetic acid). Place in an oven at $100°C$ until the spots appear. This reagent is specific for amino acids, giving a slightly different color with different amino acids.

Preparation of DNP-Protein

Dinitrofluorobenzene (DNFB) is used to detect the terminal amino acid of a free amino group (see Figures 2-1 and 2-3). This reagent reacts with all free amino groups, giving yellow compounds that are a combination of dinitrophenol (DNP) and an amino acid and are called *DNP derivatives.* Almost all DNP

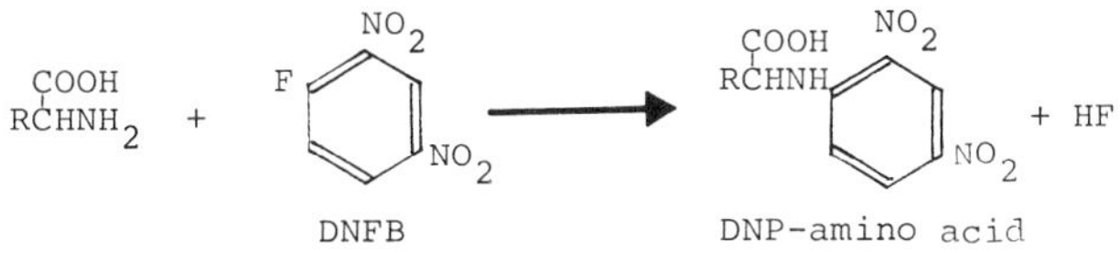

Fig. 2-3. Reaction of amino acids with dinitrofluorobenzene.

derivatives dissolve in ether, which therefore is used to extract them. DNP-arginine and DNP-lysine, however, will remain in an aqueous solution. DNP-glycine may decompose during hydrolysis, giving dinitrophenol and dinitroaniline. DNFB also reacts with the histidine and tyrosine rings, but the derivatives are colorless.

The protein is treated with DNFB and hydrolyzed by techniques described below, and the DNP—amino acid that corresponds to the terminal amino group is identified by chromatography.

Dissolve about 5 ml of the protein (or 1 mg of peptide) in 1 ml of water. Add 0.2 ml of saturated sodium bicarbonate and 2.5 ml of an ethanol solution to 10 mg/ml of dinitrofluorobenzene. Let it react for 2 hours, in the dark, shaking once in a while, and checking repeatedly to see if the pH is around 8, by taking a small drop and placing it on a pH-indicating paper. If necessary, add more bicarbonate. Lower the pH to 3 with 10 to 15 drops of 6*M* HCl, shaking while adding the acid. *Important:* Check to see that there is no open flame in the laboratory. Then add 5 ml of peroxide-free diethyl ether. Close with a clean rubber stopper and shake. Remove the ether with a dropper and repeat the procedure. This will remove the excess reagent.

Hydrolysis of DNP-Protein

Add to the sample 4.5 ml of 6*M* HCl acid, close the tube with a glass marble, and place it in the oven for five hours at $105°C$. Let it cool, and dilute it with the same amount of water. Extract three times with 5 ml ether, collecting the ether extracts in a small beaker. Let the ether evaporate and dissolve the residue with a few drops of acetone. Then transfer it to a small tube. Keep the DNP derivatives away from direct light. The ether extract will contain amino acids that have free NH_2 groups to react with DNFB. It may also contain some dinitrophenol and dinitroaniline that originate from the hydrolysis of DNP-glycine. DNP-arginine and DNP-lysine (the products of DNP with the amino group of lysine) will remain in the water phase.

Chromatography for DNP-Amino Acids

Perform thin-layer chromatography with the same plates as were used for the free amino acids. Again choose two appropriate solvents. The spots can be detected by their yellow color, or by looking at the plate in the dark under ultraviolet light (be careful not to look directly at the ultraviolet light) under which they appear as dark spots. By recording the results and comparing them, one can identify the DNP derivatives. Dinitrophenol can be recognized when the plate is exposed to hydrochloric acid fumes, since it then becomes colorless.

MOLECULAR STRUCTURE OF HEMOGLOBIN

Molecular Weight

Chemical analysis of preparations of pure hemoglobin shows that it contains 0.34 percent iron. If we assume that each molecule has only one atom of iron, the molecular weight of hemoglobin would be $56 \times 100/0.34 = 16,000$. This assumption may be checked by several methods.

The method most commonly used for the determination of the molecular weight of large molecules is ultracentrifugation. For proteins, a solution is spun in a centrifuge that provides at least 200,000 times the force of gravity and that is equipped with an optical system making it possible to observe the sedimentation of the large molecules. Measurement of the rate of sedimentation and the rate of diffusion provides data for the calculation of the molecular weight. Other methods, like light scattering and osmotic pressure, can be used also. If the molecules are very large, they can be measured under a powerful electron microscope.

A very simple method for molecular weight determination became possible with the development of Sephadex, a high molecular weight carbohydrate. This material is a molecular sieve. It comes as small beads and can be obtained with interstices of a proper size for a number of different applications. When a mixture of protein and other molecules is filtered through a column of this material, molecules smaller than the pores of Sephadex penetrate into its interstices. Those too large to penetrate are excluded and come out with the solvent. When more solvent is added to wash the column, the molecules are sorted out by their size, the larger ones coming out first.

By all these methods, hemoglobin was shown to be an almost spherical molecule of about 6.5 nm in diameter, with a molecular weight of 64,000 and containing about 10,000 atoms, four of which are iron. Hemoglobin constitutes about one-third of the total weight of the red cell.

In the presence of a high concentration of urea, a hemoglobin molecule splits into four units, each with a molecular weight of 16,000 and containing a single atom of iron. By chromatography it is possible to show that there are two types of units, called *alpha* and *beta chains.* A molecule of hemoglobin is made up of two units of each type of chain.

Heme

If a hemoglobin solution is treated with acid and acetone, as done in the preceding laboratory experiment, a colorless protein (globin) precipitates, leaving behind an acetone solution of a red compound called *hematin*, which contains all the iron of hemoglobin that in isolation is oxidized from Fe^{++} to Fe^{+++}

Hematin has been an object of investigation since 1910. Long, involved processes of classic organic chemistry, including elementary analysis, breaking the molecule through chemical reaction, and identifying the resulting products, finally led in 1929 to a structure that was confirmed by total synthesis.

As shown in Figure 2-4, *heme* is a flat molecule consisting of a large ring with conjugated double bonds and an Fe^{++} linked by ionic bonds to its center. When heme is removed from hemoglobin, the iron becomes unstable and is oxidized to Fe^{+++}.

Fig. 2-4. Heme.

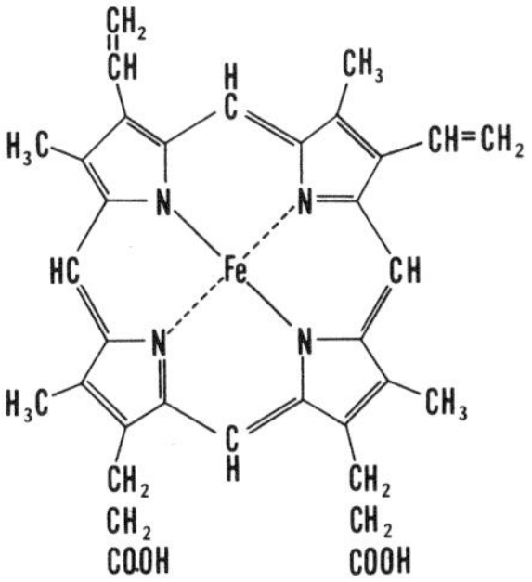

Primary Structure

Through acid hydrolysis, proteins release amino acids. Only L-isomers are present, and in neutral conditions both carboxyl and amino groups are ionized (Fig. 2-5).

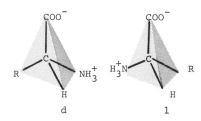

Fig. 2-5. Amino acids: D and L.

In 1906 Emil Fischer became interested in proteins. The structure of only eight amino acids was then known. Fischer isolated others, and today we know that basically proteins contain 20 different kinds of amino acids (see Fig. 2-6). Fischer found that during the hydrolysis of proteins an equal number of amino and carboxyl groups appeared. He proposed that amino acids were linked by peptide bonds. He developed methods to synthesize amino acids linked by peptide bonds — calling the amino acids thus linked *peptides* — and was able to link up to 18 amino acids.

The elucidation of the chemical structure of proteins took almost half a century after this basic observation. It was necessary first to obtain a protein in pure form, completely free of the other proteins present in living tissue. In some cases, as with insulin and hemoglobin, one gets crystals after a few simple steps of purification by precipitation with salts or organic solvents. But even crystals do not always consist of one single pure protein. Purity was only obtained after the development of physical methods like ultracentrifugation.

In the 1940s chromatography was invented, and it became a standard method of purifying and checking for purity. Using ion exchange resins (large polymers with acidic or basic groups) in column chromatography, Moore and Stein established a fast quantitative method to separate amino acids from a protein hydrolyzate. Through an automated version of this method, the 140-odd amino acids of each chain of hemoglobin were identified.

In 1945, in England, Sanger found that dinitrofluorobenzene (DNFB) reacts with the amino groups of amino acids, producing yellow compounds that can easily be identified by chromatography. Sanger treated hemoglobin with DNFB, and split the molecule through acid hydrolysis. Only one DNP-valine per chain was found (along with some DNP-ε-lysine). This showed that the chains must be long molecules of amino acids linked by peptide bonds, with

$$H_2N.CHR_1.CO-OH \quad H-NH.CHR_2.CO-OH \quad H-NH.CHR_2.CO-OH$$

$$H_2N.CHR_1.CO-HN.CHR_2.CO-HN.CHR_2.COOH$$

Fig. 2-6. Formation of peptide bonds (shaded areas).

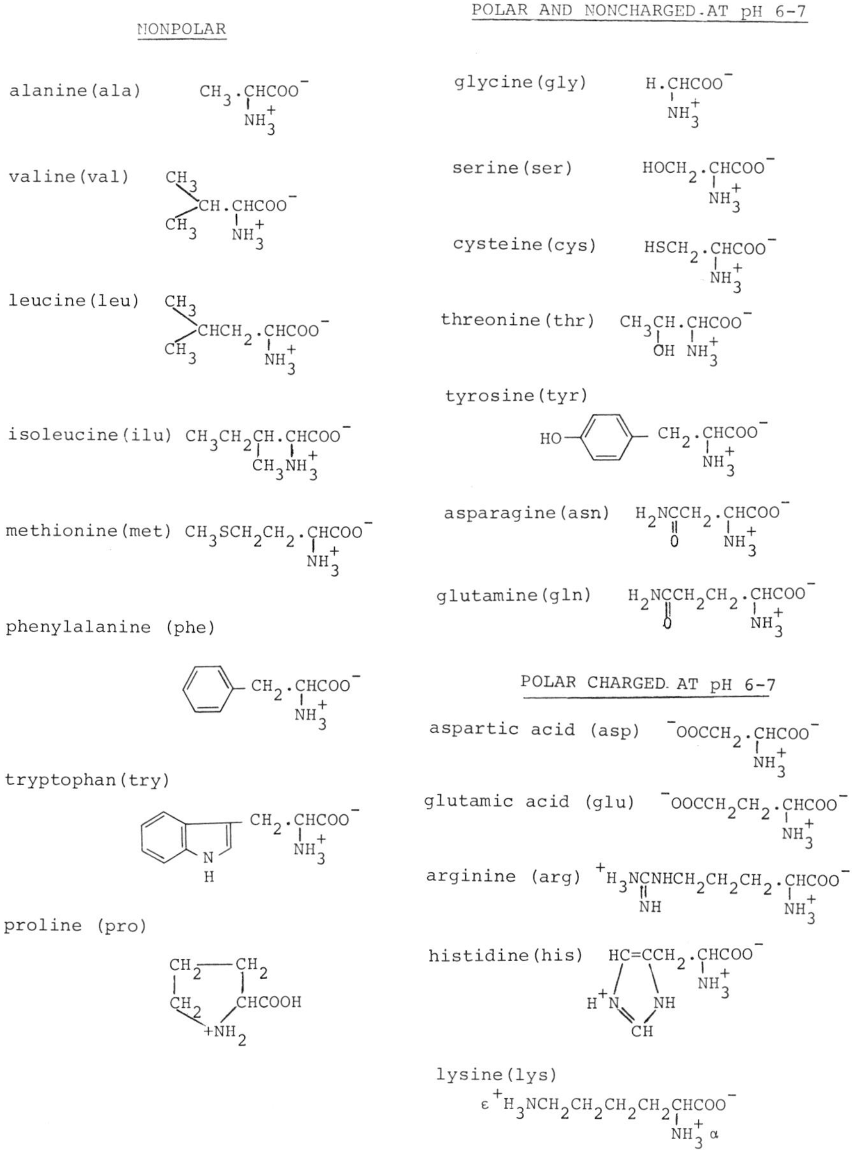

NONPOLAR

POLAR AND NONCHARGED.AT pH 6-7

alanine (ala) $CH_3 \cdot \underset{\underset{NH_3^+}{|}}{CHCOO^-}$

glycine (gly) $H \cdot \underset{\underset{NH_3^+}{|}}{CHCOO^-}$

valine (val) $\underset{CH_3}{\overset{CH_3}{>}} CH \cdot \underset{\underset{NH_3^+}{|}}{CHCOO^-}$

serine (ser) $HOCH_2 \cdot \underset{\underset{NH_3^+}{|}}{CHCOO^-}$

cysteine (cys) $HSCH_2 \cdot \underset{\underset{NH_3^+}{|}}{CHCOO^-}$

leucine (leu) $\underset{CH_3}{\overset{CH_3}{>}} CHCH_2 \cdot \underset{\underset{NH_3^+}{|}}{CHCOO^-}$

threonine (thr) $CH_3\underset{\underset{OH}{|}}{CH} \cdot \underset{\underset{NH_3^+}{|}}{CHCOO^-}$

isoleucine (ilu) $CH_3CH_2\underset{\underset{CH_3}{|}}{CH} \cdot \underset{\underset{NH_3^+}{|}}{CHCOO^-}$

tyrosine (tyr)

HO—⟨benzene ring⟩— $CH_2 \cdot \underset{\underset{NH_3^+}{|}}{CHCOO^-}$

methionine (met) $CH_3SCH_2CH_2 \cdot \underset{\underset{NH_3^+}{|}}{CHCOO^-}$

asparagine (asn) $H_2N\underset{\underset{O}{\|}}{C}CH_2 \cdot \underset{\underset{NH_3^+}{|}}{CHCOO^-}$

glutamine (gln) $H_2N\underset{\underset{O}{\|}}{C}CH_2CH_2 \cdot \underset{\underset{NH_3^+}{|}}{CHCOO^-}$

phenylalanine (phe)

⟨benzene ring⟩— $CH_2 \cdot \underset{\underset{NH_3^+}{|}}{CHCOO^-}$

POLAR CHARGED. AT pH 6-7

aspartic acid (asp) $^-OOCCH_2 \cdot \underset{\underset{NH_3^+}{|}}{CHCOO^-}$

glutamic acid (glu) $^-OOCCH_2CH_2 \cdot \underset{\underset{NH_3^+}{|}}{CHCOO^-}$

tryptophan (try)

⟨indole ring with N–H⟩— $CH_2 \cdot \underset{\underset{NH_3^+}{|}}{CHCOO^-}$

arginine (arg) $^+H_3N\underset{\underset{NH}{\|}}{C}NHCH_2CH_2CH_2 \cdot \underset{\underset{NH_3^+}{|}}{CHCOO^-}$

histidine (his) $HC=C CH_2 \cdot \underset{\underset{NH_3^+}{|}}{CHCOO^-}$ (imidazole ring)

proline (pro)

CH₂—CH₂ / CH₂ CHCOOH / ⁺NH₂ (ring structure)

lysine (lys)

$\varepsilon\,^+H_3NCH_2CH_2CH_2CH_2\underset{\underset{NH_3^+ \alpha}{|}}{CHCOO^-}$

Fig. 2-7. Amino acids present in proteins.

the last amino acid, valine, having a free amino group. The ϵ-lysine amino groups are also free; that is, they do not form peptide bonds to produce a branched molecule.

Sanger concentrated his efforts on insulin. This molecule has 777 atoms in 51 amino acids. Through acid hydrolysis he broke the insulin chains into small peptides with two to four amino acids each. Their structures were determined by the use of DNFB and by chromatographic comparison with a synthetic sample. Since the breaks occurred at random, the peptides he obtained by acid hydrolysis showed overlapping amino acids:

$$
\begin{array}{lll}
\text{Phe--Val} & \text{Asp--Glu} & \text{His--Leu} \\
\text{Val--Asp} & \text{Glu--His} & \\
\text{Phe--Val--Asp} & & \text{Leu--Cys} \\
& \text{Glu--His--Leu} & \\
\text{Val--Asp--Glu} & & \\
& & \text{His--Leu--Cys} \\
\text{Phe--Val--Asp--Glu--His} & & \\
& \text{Glu--His--Leu--Cys} &
\end{array}
$$

This led to a probable structure:

$$\text{Phe--Val--Asp--Glu--His--Leu--Cys} \ldots .$$

He also used digestive enzymes to obtain and identify more peptides. The different protein-digesting enzymes split the molecule at different points:

$$\text{R}_1 \text{ CHCO} \longrightarrow \text{NH-CHR}_2$$

The enzyme trypsin showed that R_1 must be lysine or arginine; chymotrypsin required it to be an aromatic amino acid; and pepsin required R_2 to be leucine, aspartic acid, glutamic acid, or an aromatic amino acid. He arrived at the final structure of insulin after ten years of work.

In the meantime, DuVigneau used Sanger's method to establish the structure of a much smaller molecule, oxytocin, a hormone from the pituitary gland. He was able to make a full synthetic hormone, with its eight amino acids in the proper order and with the proper configuration. He also made other, similar, polypeptides and tested their activities to find the structure requirements essential for the hormone activity.

A more convenient method was introduced later (Fig. 2-8). Phenylisothiocyanate (Erdman's reagent) reacts with the terminal amino group, and after reaction the modified amino acid can be split off, leaving the rest of the molecule intact. This terminal amino acid derivative is then identified, and the rest of the molecule treated again, until the complete sequence is established.

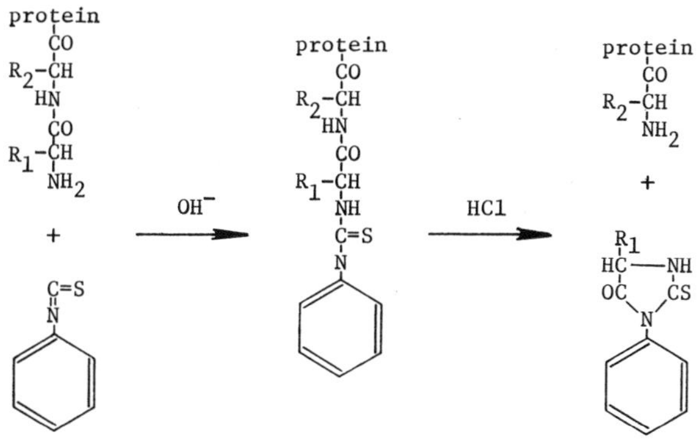

Fig. 2-8. Erdman's method for amino acid sequencing. Left, phenylisothio-cyanate; right, phenylthiohidantoin.

Using these various methods, by 1961 several groups of investigators (Braunitzer, Konigsberg, Hill, Schroeder) established the structure of hemoglobin chain and of the single chain of myoglobin, a protein that exists in muscles. Each of these chains contains a sequence of about 140 amino acids (Table 2-2).

The sequence of amino acids of many proteins has now been established, and laboratories continue to analyze new proteins. Although some proteins are built of more than one chain, in all cases the chain is a linear polymer, consisting of a sequence of amino acids linked by peptide bonds. In each position in the chain there may be any one of twenty different amino acids, giving a total of 10^{184} different possible structures the same size as a hemoglobin chain. If there were one molecule of each of these, the resulting mass would be about 2×10^{165} g. In comparison, the mass of the earth is only 6×10^{27} g and the total matter in the universe is 2×10^{55} g!

Comparing hemoglobin chains present in different species with those in humans one finds the following amino acid differences:

Species	Alpha Chain	Beta Chain
monkey	4	8
horse	18	26
cow	17	26
rabbit	25	14
kangaroo	24	38
chicken	35	....
carp	71	....

These differences occur when one amino acid is replaced by another or is just missing entirely.

Table 2-2. Primary Structure of Myoglobin and Hemoglobin Chains

	Man					Horse	
	myo	α	β	γ	δ	α	β
NA1	gly	val	val	gly	val	val	val
2		his	his	his			gln
3	leu	leu	leu	phe	leu	leu	leu
A1	ser	ser	thr	thr	thr	ser	ser
A2	asp	pro	pro	glu	pro	ala	gly
3	gly	ala	glu	glu	glu	ala	glu
4	glu	asp	glu	asp	glu	asp	glu
5	trp	lys	lys	lys	lys	lys	lys
6	gln	thr	ser	ala	thr	thr	ala
7	leu	asn	ala	thr	ala	asn	ala
8	val	val	val	ilu	val	val	val
9	leu	lys	thr	thr	asn	lys	leu
10	asn	ala	ala	ser	ala	ala	ala
11	val	ala	leu	leu	leu	ala	leu
12	trp	trp	trp	trp	trp	trp	trp
13	gly	gly	gly	gly	gly	ser	asp
14	lys	lys	lys	lys	lys	lys	lys
15	val	val	val	val	val	val	val
16	glu	gly	asn	asn	asn	gly	asn
AB1	ilu	ala				gly	
B1	asp	his				his	
2	val	ala	val	val	val	ala	glu
3	ala	gly	asp	glu	asp	gly	glu
4	gly	glu	glu	asp	ala	glu	glu
5	his	tyr	val	ala	val	tyr	val
6	gly	gly	gly	gly	gly	gly	gly
7	glu	ala	gly	gly	gly	ala	gly
8	glu	glu	glu	glu	glu	glu	glu
9	val	ala	ala	thr	ala	ala	ala
10	leu	leu	leu	leu	leu	leu	leu
11	phe	glu	gly	gly	gly	glu	gly
12	lys	arg	arg	arg	arg	arg	arg
13	gly	met	leu	leu	leu	met	leu
14	his	phe	leu	leu	leu	phe	leu
15	pro	leu	val	val	val	leu	val
16	lys	ser	val	val	val	gly	val
C1	thr	phe	tyr	tyr	tyr	phe	tyr
2	lys	pro	pro	pro	pro	pro	pro
3	phe	thr	trp	trp	trp	thr	trp
4	asp	thr	thr	thr	thr	thr	thr
5	arg	lys	gln	gln	gln	lys	gln
6	phe	thr	arg	arg	arg	thr	arg
7	lys	tyr	phe	phe	phe	tyr	phe
CD1	phe	phe	phe	phe	phe	phe	phe
2	asp	pro	glu	asp	glu	pro	asp
3	arg	his	ser	ser	ser	his	ser
4	phe	phe	phe	phe	phe	phe	phe
5	lys		gly	gly	gly		gly
6	his	asp	asp	asn	asp	asp	asp
7	leu	leu	leu	leu	leu	leu	leu
8	lys	ser	ser	ser	ser	ser	ser
D1	ser	his	thr	ser	ser	his	gly
2	glu		pro	ala	pro		pro
3	asp		asp	ser	asp		asp
4	glu		ala	ala	ala		ala
5	met		val	ilu	val		val
6	lys		met	met	met		met
7	ala	gly	gly	gly	gly	gly	gly
E1	ser	ser	asn	asn	asn	ser	asn
2	glu	ala	pro	pro	pro	ala	pro
3	asp	gln	lys	lys	lys	gln	lys
4	leu	val	val	val	val	val	val
5	lys	lys	lys	lys	lys	lys	lys
6	lys	gly	ala	ala	ala	ala	ala
7	his	his	his	his	his	his	his
8	gly	gly	gly	gly	gly	gly	gly
9	ala	lys	lys	lys	lys	lys	lys
10	thr	lys	lys	lys	lys	lys	lys
11	val	val	val	val	val	val	val
12	leu	ala	leu	leu	leu	ala	leu
13	thr	asp	gly	thr	gly	asp	his
14	ala	ala	ala	ser	ala	gly	ser
15	leu	leu	phe	leu	phe	leu	phe
16	gly	thr	ser	gly	ser	thr	gly
17	gly	asn	asp	asp	asp	leu	glu
18	ilu	ala	gly	ala	gly	ala	gly
19	leu	val	leu	ilu	leu	val	val
20	lys	ala	ala	lys	ala	gly	his
EF1	lys	his	his	his	his	his	his
2	lys	val	leu	leu	leu	leu	leu
3	gly	asp	asp	asp	asp	asp	asp
4	his	asp	asn	asp	asn	asp	asn
5	his	met	leu	leu	leu	leu	leu
6	glu	pro	lys	lys	lys	pro	lys
7	ala	asn	gly	gly	gly	gly	gly
8	glu	ala	thr	thr	thr	ala	thr

Table 2-2.   (Cont.)

	Man				Horse			Man				Horse	
	myo	α	β	γ	δ	α	β		myo	α	β	γ	δ	α	β
F1	ilu	leu	phe	phe	phe	leu	phe	GH1	his	leu	phe	phe	phe	leu	phe
2	lys	ser	ala	ala	ser	ser	ala	2	pro	pro	gly	gly	gly	pro	gly
3	pro	ala	thr	gln	gln	asp	ala	3	gly	ala	lys	lys	lys	asn	lys
4	leu	leu	leu	leu	leu	leu	leu	4	asn	glu	glu	glu	glu	asp	asp
5	ala	ser	ser	ser	ser	ser	ser	5	phe	phe	phe	phe	phe	phe	phe
6	gln	asp	glu	glu	glu	asn	glu	6	gly	thr	thr	thr	thr	thr	thr
7	ser	leu	leu	leu	leu	leu	leu	H1	ala	pro	pro	pro	pro	pro	pro
8	his	his	his	his	his	his	his	2	asp	ala	pro	glu	gln	ala	glu
9	ala	ala	cys	cys	cys	ala	cys	3	ala	val	val	val	met	val	leu
FG1	thr	his	asp	asp	asp	his	asp	4	gln	his	gln	gln	gln	his	gln
2	lys	lys	lys	lys	lys	lys	lys	5	gly	ala	ala	ala	ala	ala	ala
3	his	leu	leu	leu	leu	leu	leu	6	ala	ser	ala	ser	ala	ser	ser
4	lys	arg	his	his	his	arg	his	7	met	leu	tyr	trp	tyr	leu	tyr
5	val	val	val	val	val	val	val	8	asn	asp	gln	gln	gln	asp	gln
G1	pro	asp	asp	asp	asp	asp	asp	9	lys	lys	lys	lys	lys	lys	lys
2	ilu	pro	pro	pro	pro	pro	pro	10	ala	phe	val	met	val	phe	val
3	lys	val	glu	glu	glu	val	glu	11	leu	leu	val	val	val	leu	val
4	tyr	asn	asn	asn	asn	asn	asn	12	glu	ala	ala	thr	ala	ser	ala
5	leu	phe	phe	phe	phe	phe	phe	13	leu	ser	gly	gly	gly	ser	gly
6	glu	lys	arg	lys	arg	lys	arg	14	phe	val	val	val	val	val	val
7	phe	leu	leu	leu	leu	leu	leu	15	arg	ser	ala	ala	ala	ser	ala
8	ilu	leu	leu	leu	leu	leu	leu	16	lys	thr	asn	ser	asn	thr	asn
9	ser	ser	gly	gly	gly	ser	gly	17	asp	val	ala	ala	ala	val	ala
10	glu	his	asn	asn	asn	his	asn	18	met	leu	leu	leu	leu	leu	leu
11	cys	cys	val	val	val	cys	val	19	ala	thr	ala	ser	ala	thr	ala
12	ilu	leu	leu	leu	leu	leu	leu	20	ser	ser	his	ser	his	ser	his
13	ilu	leu	val	val	val	leu	ala	21	asn	lys	lys	arg	lys	lys	lys
14	gln	val	cys	thr	cys	ser	leu	22	tyr	tyr	tyr	tyr	tyr	tyr	tyr
15	val	thr	val	val	val	thr	val	23	lys	arg	his	his	his	arg	his
16	leu	leu	leu	leu	leu	leu	val	24	glu						
17	gln	ala	ala	ala	ala	ala	ala	HI1	leu						
18	ser	ala	his	ilu	arg	val	arg	2	gly						
19	lys	his	his	his	asn	his	his	3	phe						
								4	gln						
								5	gly						

Most of human adult hemoglobin is hemoglobin A, with two alpha and two beta chains. About 2 percent is hemoglobin A_2, with two alpha and two delta chains. During fetal life and in the newborn, fetal hemoglobin exists, with two alpha and two gamma chains. In the first three months of fetal life, a fourth hemoglobin exists, called Gower I. This contains two alpha and two epsilon chains. The structures of the epsilon chains are not yet known.

The similarity of hemoglobin and myoglobin chains in different species allows us to build an evolutionary tree that coincides with that based on other biological data and suggests that it took about 10 million years for the establishment of a single amino acid change for hemoglobin. On the basis of this we can imagine that there was initially a single chain, as exists for lamprey hemoglobin, and that after about 650 million years myoglobin and the alpha chain of hemoglobin originated from this primitive chain. Three hundred fifty million years ago the alpha chain gave rise to the beta chain. The gamma chain must have appeared about 150 million years ago, and the delta only 35 million years ago.

Although there are quite a large number of polypeptide chains with the same amino acid composition as insulin, in 1964 Katzoyanis in the United States and Wang in China were able to obtain the proper sequence and to produce synthetic insulin. Their original long, tedious chemical process has now been replaced by a technique introduced by Merrifield (Fig. 2-9). An amino

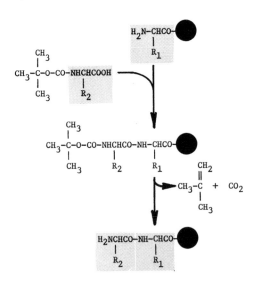

Fig. 2-9. Merrifield's method for polypeptide synthesis.

acid is combined with a special resin. A derivative of the next amino acid, with the amino group blocked, is then added, and reacts to form a dipeptide. The process continues in this manner, and it is possible to add amino acids stepwise to produce a synthetic protein. Recently, growth hormone, with its 188 amino acids, was made by Merrifield's method.

Tridimensional Structure

One of Pauling's earlier and more important contributions came from his studies of water. In a molecule of water, the electrons are strongly attracted by the oxygen, which is negative in relation to the hydrogen atoms, creating a permanent electric dipole. The oxygen of one molecule has a weak attractive force on the hydrogen of other molecules, and this attraction forms what is commonly known as a *hydrogen bond* (Fig. 2-10). In ice, there are many

Fig. 2-10. A. Water molecule, showing charges. B. Hydrogen bonds (dotted lines) between water molecules.

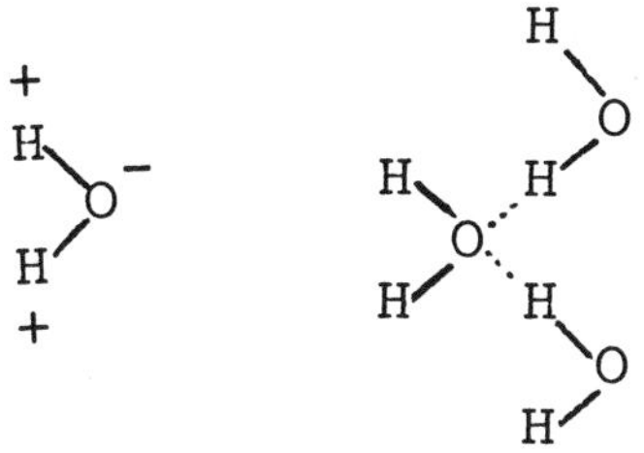

hydrogen bonds, which create a crystalline structure. Some of the bonds break on melting. Hydrogen bonds can be formed between other groups with permanent dipoles, such as $C=O \ldots HO$ or $C=O \ldots HN$.

In the beginning of this century it was discovered by Bragg, in England, that when x-rays hit a crystal they become scattered. The reflected x-ray waves interfere with each other, adding or subtracting according to their phase. A film registers the pattern of this addition and subtraction as a number of spots. The process of scattering and interference is in every respect similar to what happens to the light going through a slide when you examine an object under the microscope. Unfortunately there is no optical device that can reform the image so that one can see it. The only possibility is to use the spots to reconstruct the image. This is similar to trying to reconstruct the position of the piles of a dock by using their reflection in the image of the water waves hitting them. One has as data the intensity of the spots, but there is no way to record on film the phase of the waves.

With simple molecules, one can propose a probable structure, analyze the data, and by successive approximations correct the proposed model. This is a lot more difficult with large molecules and with structures that are not as regular as inorganic crystals. It is seen that n atoms give n^2 reflections. Therefore, it is much easier if one can recognize a part of the molecule. Heavy metals can be introduced within a molecule at specific points and can be easily recognized by x-ray interference patterns, since they scatter more intensively than light atoms. Computerized methods today allow one to examine a very large number of spots and through this to determine large structures. In the 1930s Austbury used x-ray diffraction to examine hair, Bernal began to work on proteins, and Perutz and Kendrew started to study hemoglobin and myoglobin. Yet it took until the end of the fifties for them to reconstruct those molecules. Through computation of more and more reflected spots, resolution was improved, and today the data on myoglobin is accurate to 15 nm, which means essentially that all atoms have been located.

Physical methods show that proteins are not the very long, linear chains that the primary structure might suggest. Actually the hemoglobin molecule is spherical. A major development was introduced by Pauling and Corey in 1951 when they reported on their investigation with x-ray diffraction, comparing simple synthetic peptides to proteins. They were able to establish that the six atoms of the peptide bond must lie in a plane, as had been foreseen from the sharing of a double bond by C–C and by C–N (Fig. 2-11). They also found that

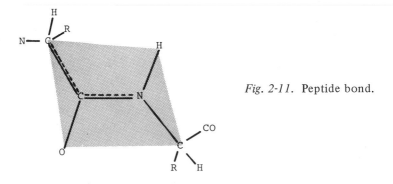

Fig. 2-11. Peptide bond.

their data fitted a model structure called the *alpha helix,* in which the polypeptide chain is twisted in a helical shape, each turn consisting of 13 atoms from 3.6 amino acids (Fig. 2-12). The hydrogen atom of an NH group is attracted to the oxygen atom of a C=O group, forming a hydrogen bond

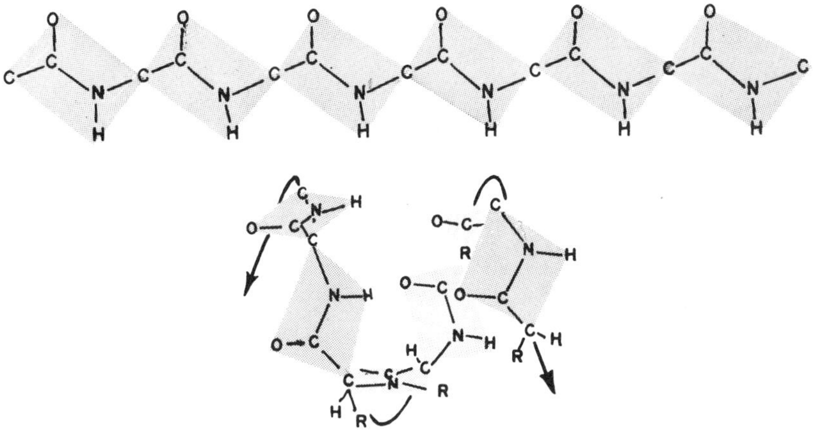

Fig. 2-12. Formation of an alpha helix. Top, the peptide chain; bottom, in helical formation.

(Fig. 2-13). Such a helical structure would have the property of changing the plane of polarized light. This is independent of the asymmetrical carbons. It is demonstrated in the case of polyglycine, in which the alpha carbon is not an asymmetrical carbon and does not have side chains.

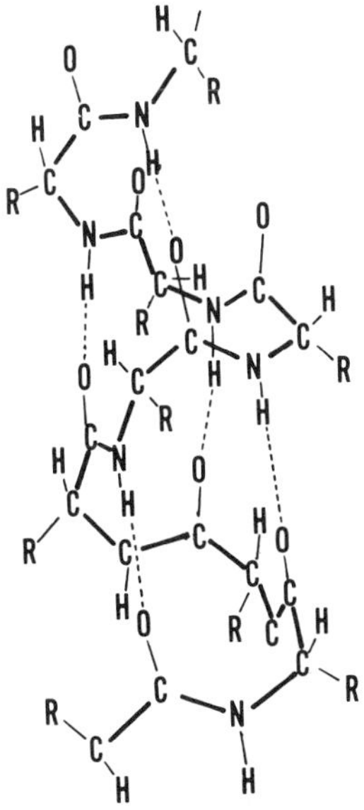

Fig. 2-13. Alpha helix showing hydrogen bonds.

Because proteins have L-amino acids, a right-hand helix accommodates the amino acid side chains best. Proline, however, does not fit the alpha helix structure. Here the amino acid has a rigid ring structure and is missing the hydrogen for the hydrogen bond. Also, one would expect that the proximity of several side chains with similar charges (e.g., ionized carboxyl groups of aspartic and glutamic acids, or epsilon amino groups of lysine and arginine) would disrupt the structure because of electrical repulsions.

Remember that the usual chemical formula of alanine as shown by the common stick and ball model has quite a lot of empty space. Models that show the space filled by each atom provide a much more compact structure (Fig. 2-14).[*]

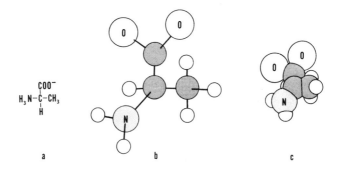

Fig. 2-14. Structure of an amino acid. (a) structural formula, (b) stick and ball model showing bond angles, (c) Stuart space-filling model showing space occupied by the atoms.

An amazingly similar pattern was discovered in myoglobin and hemoglobin chains from vertebrates, hemoglobin chains from the lamprey, and even chains from invertebrates. These all have the same general shape. At certain points, in many cases due to the existence of proline, there are bends in the molecule, shaping it in a very compact spherical structure, with room for about four molecules of water. The straight segments have an alpha helix structure. (See Figure 2-15).

Examining the structure of proteins led to the discovery of another important feature. Due to ionized groups, or displaced electrons, some amino acid

---

[*]A good idea of the tridimensional structure of myoglobin is given by the computer-generated film *Myoglobin* (K. R. Wilson, Harper and Row, sound film or loop). The data obtained from crystallography is transformed into symbols representing a tridimensional structure that is turned to show how it looks from different angles.

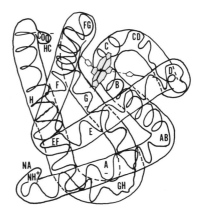

Fig. 2-15. Myoglobin. Amino acid sequence for each segment is shown in Figure 2-9.

side chains have a permanent electric dipole, similar to that of water. These *polar groups* interact with water and are therefore water soluble. In the hemoglobin and myoglobin molecules one finds polar groups facing outward as would be expected, surrounded by a layer of immobilized water molecules.

Other groups, with only hydrogen and carbon atoms, are *nonpolar.* They do not interact with water, but disturb the water structure. They tend to withdraw from water, coming together and being held by very weak short-range forces known as *van der Waals forces.* These are found in the inside of the protein molecule, and lead to packing of the groups.

The tridimensional structure is essentially the consequence of the interaction of polar and nonpolar groups, which tend to build an equilibrated structure by folding the chain. This allows for further interaction between side chains at different points of the molecule, either through hydrogen bonding or through ionic attraction.

The stability of the tridimensional structure depends on all these interactions. If one cut the myoglobin molecule into segments having an alpha helix structure, they would not remain helical, as hydrogen bonds alone are not sufficient to keep such a structure intact.

A number of substances — e.g., urea and guanidine — through mechanisms such as disturbing water structure, forming hydrogen bonds, and disturbing nonpolar group interactions, will destroy both the alpha helix (secondary) and the spatial conformation (tertiary structure), and the polypeptide chain will fold randomly. This is called *denaturation,* and it results in a change of the biological and physicochemical properties of the molecule. Frequently the denatured protein is insoluble. On denaturation there is a decrease in the rotation of polarized light due to the unwinding of the alpha helix. Hydrogens that have been either inside the molecule or bound by hydrogen bonds now become accessible and can be interchanged with deuterium when the molecule is suspended in heavy water. Chemical groups which might have different properties when inside a protein molecule (away from water and in a medium with different properties) return to normal (e.g., the strength of acidic and basic groups changes and cysteine SH groups which in native protein do not react chemically become reactive).

If denaturation is not too harsh, that is, if covalent bonds are not broken, returning the protein to normal conditions may cause it to be slowly *renatured,* that is, to revert to its original structure. This is the most stable structure under normal or cellular conditions.

In the middle of the most compact structure of hemoglobin there is a pocket lined by nonpolar side chains, which the flat heme group occupies (Fig. 2-17).*
The heme is bound to the protein by a coordinate bond between the iron in heme and one of the histidine residues, F^8, in globin, that supplies two electrons to the iron. In this protective environment, in which there is room for only one

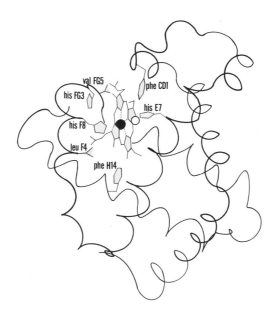

Fig. 2-16. Amino acid pocket around heme. The black circle represents the iron atom.

*With the help of a stereo viewer a tridimensional representation of the groups surrounding the heme may be seen in *Nature* 219:907 (1968).

molecule of water, iron remains in its ferrous form (Fe^{++}), not oxidizing to ferric even with the introduction of an oxygen molecule as blood passes through the lungs.

It is amazing that the structure of hemoglobins and myoglobins is so similar, considering that they have only seven amino acids in common. Four are in close contact with the heme; one of these is the histidine F^8 bonded to the heme iron; a second histidine, F^7, is bonded to the iron through water. The leucine is important in that it seems to place the first histidine in position in relation to the heme, and the phenylalanine seems to play a specific role, lining up parallel to heme with its double bonds overlapping the heme double bonds.

All substitutions of one amino acid for another that occur in myoglobin and hemoglobin in any species must occur in a way that is compatible with preserving the general structure and function of these two molecules.

Quarternary Structure: Assembling the Molecule

Each hemoglobin has two alpha and two beta chains. The assembly of the protein molecule with two or more chains is called the quarternary structure.

The chains occupy positions resembling the corners of a tetrahedron (Fig. 2-17), and are held together by weak bonds, specifically nonpolar group

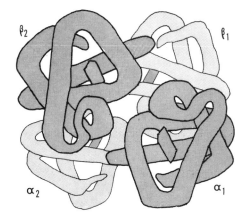

Fig. 2-17. Spatial position of the four chains of hemoglobin.

interactions. As with myoglobin, nonpolar groups replace polar groups to create the interface that brings the chains together, leaving a channel about 200 nm wide between chains.

LABORATORY INVESTIGATION: PROPERTIES OF HEMOGLOBIN

1. Amino acids have basic and acidic groups. Titrate 10 ml of 0.1*M* glycine with 0.1*M* hydrochloric acid and with 0.1*M* sodium hydroxide. (For background information and measurement of pH see Appendix V; pH, Titration, and Buffers.) After the addition of aliquots of 1 ml, measure the pH and plot it against the amount of acid or base added. Repeat the titration, replacing the glycine with (a) plain distilled water, (b) acetic acid, and (c) methylamine (see Figure 2-18).

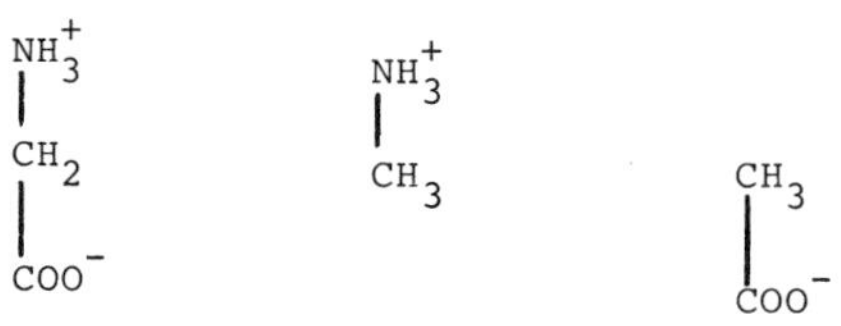

$$\overset{+}{NH_3}-CH_2-COO^-$$

$$\overset{+}{NH_3}-CH_3$$

$$CH_3-COO^-$$

Fig. 2-18. Glycine and related compounds. Left, glycine; center, methylamine; right, acetic acid.

Find out if the solutions used are buffers and, if so, in what range of pH. Calculate the pK, and, by comparing the three compounds, the groups being titrated.

2. Study the buffer capacity of hemoglobin and oxyhemoglobin, and find out if they are the same.

3. Hemoglobin has a characteristic absorption spectrum. Use a spectrophotometer to measure the absorption of light at different wavelengths between 400 and 700 nm (at intervals of 25 nm). Plot the results to obtain a characteristic absorption spectrum. Investigate to see if this spectrum changes when (a) oxygen, (b) carbon dioxide, and (c) carbon monoxide are bubbled into the hemoglobin solution. Find out if you can displace one gas with the other.

Procedures

Use a red cell hemolyzate as a source of hemoglobin. All oxygen may be removed (both that contained in hemoglobin and that dissolved in the solution) by adding a small amount of sodium dithionate. Introduce each gas in turn by bubbling it through a fine pipette. Use air as a source of oxygen. Carbon dioxide may be produced by causing hydrochloric acid to react with a bicarbonate, and carbon monoxide by adding to 5 ml of concentrated formic acid about 1 ml of concentrated sulfuric acid.

PHYSIOLOGICAL ROLE OF HEMOGLOBIN

Transport of Oxygen

An average man, seated, uses about 600 cm^3 of oxygen each minute. He removes this from an amount of air 20 times that volume by pumping it in and out of his lungs. This air is exposed to the blood on a surface of 100 m^2 inside the lungs. The total volume of blood passing through the lungs is at least 15 thousand liters per day!

Even this huge volume cannot carry more than a small percentage of dissolved oxygen compared to what the body needs. However, while traveling through the lungs (the total time span being about half a second), the molecules of hemoglobin of each red cell combine with oxygen. This accounts for the full transport of oxygen between lung and tissue.

Oxygen combines with the iron of the heme group in a reversible reaction. At the lungs, where there is a high concentration of oxygen (equivalent to a partial pressure of 105 mm Hg), oxyhemoglobin is formed, and at the tissues, where the concentration of oxygen is lower (equivalent to 40 mm Hg), it decomposes, releasing oxygen.

As shown by Figure 2-19, myoglobin has a higher affinity for oxygen than does hemoglobin and so can remove the oxygen from the blood and store it

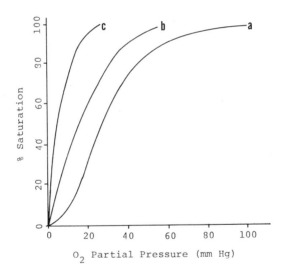

Fig. 2-19. Saturation curves for (a) hemoglobin, (b) myoglobin, and (c) cytochrome oxidase.

inside the muscle cell. In the mitochondria there is another iron-containing pigment, cytochrome oxidase, which is responsible for the use of oxygen during cell respiration. It has a much higher affinity for oxygen than has hemoglobin or myoglobin. Fetal hemoglobin also has a higher affinity for oxygen than has hemoglobin of the adult. This is responsible for the transfer of oxygen from maternal blood to the fetus, and protects the fetus from asphyxia.

There is a major difference in the shape of the affinity curve for oxygen between myoglobin and hemoglobin. The S-shaped hemoglobin curve (Fig. 2-20) indicates that each heme does not behave independently of the

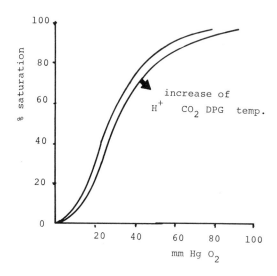

Fig. 2-20. Bohr effect.

other heme groups in the same molecule. It becomes successively easier to make hemoglobin react with one, two, three and four oxygens. Moreover, the curve is displaced to the right when the pH is lowered or CO_2 concentration is increased; this is called the *Bohr effect.* All this contributes to make hemoglobin release oxygen at the level of the tissues, where the O_2 and pH levels are lower and the CO_2 level higher. The reverse occurs in the lung.

This shift to the right of the oxyhemoglobin dissociation curve also occurs when 2-3 diphosphoglyceric acid (DPG) is added. This is a metabolite of the glucose metabolism in the red cell, and exists in high concentrations. It enters the groove between the hemoglobin chains that bind one molecule to the two N-terminal amino groups of the beta chains, and competes with oxygen, displacing it. The concentration of DPG increases during anaerobiosis, and cooperates with the increase of hydrogen ions and carbon dioxide to split oxyhemoglobin, providing the cells with more oxygen.

In people living at high altitudes, the blood hemoglobin content is increased to compensate for the low oxygen pressure. The hemoglobin dissociation curve also presents a shift to the right which seems to result from a higher level of DPG.

The same right shift occurs at higher than normal temperatures, and provides a mechanism for faster oxygen supply to the tissues during fever.

Carbon monoxide has a very high affinity for hemoglobin and myoglobin: 200 times stronger than that of oxygen. When the reaction takes place, a stable compound is formed. That is the explanation for the toxicity of this gas.

It has long been known that hemoglobin and oxyhemoglobin crystallize in different forms and therefore must have different molecular shapes. Perutz found that when oxygen combines with the hemoglobin molecule, the two alpha chains, and even more, the two beta chains, move closer together, opening again when oxygen is released. In 1936 Pauling studied the magnetic properties of hemoglobin and oxyhemoglobin. He found that hemoglobin is paramagnetic, with the four unpaired iron electrons bound by ionic forces to the heme groups. On oxygenation, there is a change in the distribution of the electrons, and they pair, producing a diamagnetic molecule whose iron is bound to the heme by covalent bonds (Fig. 2-21).

Only recently a more detailed picture of the transformation of hemoglobin to oxyhemoglobin was established by the use of x-ray diffraction. This revealed how complex the molecule really is.

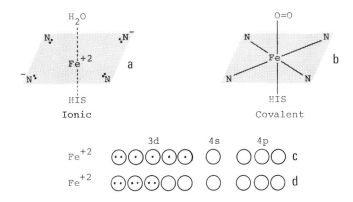

Fig. 2-21. Bond structure of heme in (a) hemoglobin and (b) oxyhemoglobin, showing the related electronic configuration of the iron atoms in the (c) ionic and (d) covalent compounds.

The change in the electronic configuration results in a change in the diameter of the iron atom. On combining with oxygen, the iron no longer fits the plane of the heme ring, and moves out toward histidine F^8. This triggers a change in the tertiary structure of the chain, breaking the hydrogen bond between tyrosine H^{22} and valine FG^5 (Fig. 2-16). The two halves of the hemoglobin molecule, each with one alpha and one beta chain, rotate in opposite directions and move apart. The ionic bond between the terminal carboxyl amino acids (arginine of alpha 1 and histidine of beta 1) breaks. The histidine ionizes, releasing hydrogen ions and making oxyhemoglobin a stronger acid than hemoglobin. Increasing hydrogen ion concentration and lowering oxygen concentration reverses the changes, dissociating the oxyhemoglobin.

Transport of Carbon Dioxide

Table 2-3. Transport of Carbon Dioxide in Blood

Form of CO_2	In Arterial Blood	In Venous Blood	A-V Difference
Plasma CO_2	0.71	0.80	+0.09
Plasma HCO_3^-	15.23	16.19	+0.96
Total plasma	15.94	16.99	+1.05
Red cell CO_2	0.34	0.39	+0.05
Red cell HCO_3^-	4.28	4.41	+0.13
Red cell carbamino-hemoglobin	0.97	1.42	+0.45
Total red cell	5.59	6.62	+0.63
Total CO_2	1.05	1.19	+0.14
Total HCO_3^-	19.51	20.60	+1.09
Total red cell carbamino-hemoglobin	0.97	1.42	+0.45
Total	21.53	23.21	+1.68

Examining Table 2-3, one can see that the major part of carbon dioxide in blood is transported as plasma bicarbonate. Red cells play a fundamental role in this process. The reaction of carbon dioxide with water, which normally is very slow, is accelerated by an enzyme (carbonic anhydrase) contained within the red cell. The bicarbonate ions then diffuse to the plasma:

$$CO_2 + H_2O \rightleftharpoons HCO_2^- + H^+$$

Apparently hemoglobin carries out only a small part of the transport of CO_2, in the form of carbamino groups:

$$HbO_2 - NH_2 + CO_2 \rightleftharpoons Hb - NHCOO^- + H^+$$

However, the hemoglobin molecule is indispensable to most of the transport of CO_2 in that it acts as a buffer. It takes up 1.45 of the 1.54 hydrogen ions produced during the oxyhemoglobin-to-hemoglobin reaction and during the formation of carbamino groups. The serum proteins buffer part of the rest, and the result is a very small pH change, which is compatible with life.

SELF-EVALUATION

1. A polypeptide was analyzed, and it was found
   that by acid hydrolysis it contained Ala, Arg, His, Leu, and Phe;
   that by treatment with DNFB, followed by hydrolysis and ether extraction, DNP-ala was isolated;
   that by trypsin digestion it produced two peptides, one tripeptide containing ala, arg, and phe, and another containing his, leu, and phe;
   that when this second peptide was treated by DNFB, no ether-soluble DNP—amino acid was produced;
   that treatment of this second peptide with chymotrypsin released leucine;
   that treatment of the polypeptide with chymotrypsin produced ala—phe, leu, and a peptide containing arg, his, leu, and phe.
Write the primary structure of this polypeptide.

2. The iron in hemoglobin reacts
   a. with oxygen only.
   b. with oxygen and carbon dioxide.
   c. with oxygen and carbon monoxide.
   d. with all three gases.

3. Denaturation is
   a. a change in protein properties due to a change in the tridimensional structure.
   b. a change in protein properties due to a modification in the primary structure.
   c. a change in protein properties due to breaking of peptide bonds.
   d. none of the above.

4. Carbon dioxide is transported
   a. mainly as dissolved carbon dioxide.
   b. mainly as dissolved bicarbonate in the serum.
   c. mainly as dissolved bicarbonate in the red cells.
   d. mainly combined to hemoglobin.

5. The Bohr effect is
   a. changes in the electronic structure of iron.
   b. the effect of pH and carbon dioxide on the dissociation of oxyhemo-globin.
   c. the reversible dissociation of oxyhemoglobin.
   d. the inactivation of hemoglobin by carbon monoxide.

6. The sigmoid shape of the dissociation curve of oxyhemoglobin shows
   a. heme-heme interaction.
   b. that removal of oxygen from the red cells is more difficult than from a solution of hemoglobin.
   c. properties similar to all oxygen carriers.
   d. more dissociation of oxyhemoglobin at a higher concentration of oxygen.

7. To check if a person died of asphyxia due to carbon monoxide one should
   a. measure the amount of hemoglobin iron.
   b. measure the total amount of hemoglobin.
   c. do a hematocrit.
   d. make a spectral curve of hemolyzed blood.

8. When titrating an amino acid with acid, one
   a. titrates the amino groups.
   b. titrates the carboxyl groups.
   c. titrates both the carboxyl and the amino groups.

FURTHER READINGS

Antonini, E., and Brunori, M. Hemoglobin. *Ann. Rev. Biochem.* 39:977, 1970.

Bailey, J. L. *Techniques in Protein Chemistry.* 2nd ed. Amsterdam: Elsevier, 1967.

Blackburn, S. *Protein Sequence Determination.* New York: Dekker, 1970.

Braunitzer, G., et al. *Adv. Protein Chem.* Vol. 19, 1964.

Bryason, V., and Vogel, H. J. (Eds.) *Evolving Genes and Proteins.* New York: Academic, 1965.

Dayhoff, M. O., and Eck, R. V. *Atlas of Protein Sequence.* Washington, D. C.: National Biomedical Research, 1969.

Dickerson, R. E., and Geis, I. *The Structure and Action of Proteins.* New York: Harper & Row, 1969.

Edman, P. A protein sequenator. *Eur. J. Biochem.* 1:80, 1967.

Fitch, W. M., and Margliash, E. Construction of phylogenetic trees. *Science* 155:279, 1967.

Fraenkel-Conrad, H., Harris, J. I., and Levy, A. L. Recent developments in techniques for terminal and sequence studies in peptides and proteins. *Methods Biochem. Anal.* 2:359, 1955.

Harkness, D. R. The regulation of hemoglobin oxygenation. *Adv. Intern. Med.* 17:189, 1972.

Holmes, K. C., and Blow, D. M. *The Use of X-ray Diffraction in the Study of Protein and Nucleic Acid Structure.* Baltimore, Md.: Interscience, 1965.

Katsoyanis, P. G. The synthesis of insulin. *Recent Prog. Horm. Res.* 23:505, 1967.

Katsoyanis, P. G., and Ginos, J. Z. Chemical synthesis of peptides. *Ann. Rev. Biochem.* 38:881, 1969.

Merrifield, R. B. Automated synthesis of peptides. *Science* 150:178, 1965.

Needleman, S. B. (Ed.) *Protein Sequence Determination.* Berlin: Springer, 1970.

Neurath, J. (Ed.) *The Proteins* (2nd ed.). 4 vols. New York: Academic, 1964.

Neiderwasser, A., and Tataki, G. *New Techniques in Amino Acids, Peptides and Protein Analysis.* Ann Arbor, Mich.: Ann Arbor Science, 1971.

Pauling, L., and Corey, R. B. Configurations of polypeptide chains with favored orientations around single bonds: two new pleated sheets. *Proc. Natl. Acad. Sci.* 37:729, 1951.

Pauling, L., Corey, R. B., and Branson, H. R. The structure of proteins: two hydrogen-bonded helical configurations of the polypeptide chain. *Proc. Natl. Acad. Sci.* 37:205, 1951.

Pertuz, M. F., and Lehmann, H. Molecular Pathology of human hemoglobin . Nature 219:902, 1969.

Sanger, F., and Thompson Teha, E. O. P. Amino acid sequence of the glycine chain of insulin. *Biochem. J.* 53:353, 1963.

Sanger, F., and Tuppy, H. The amino acid sequence in the phenylalanine chain of insulin. *Biochem. J.* 49:463, 1951.

Structure and function of proteins at the three-dimensional level. Cold Spring Harbor Symposia. *Quantitative Biology* Vol. 26, 1972.

Yon, J. *Structure et dynamique conformationnelle des proteines.* Paris: Herman, 1969.

3 From Molecules to Disease: Anemias

STUDY GUIDE

On the basis of what the first two chapters have established about red cells and hemoglobin, their relationship to disease will now be explored. This chapter should enable you to do the following:

1. Understand that anemia corresponds to a decrease in red cell population and/or hemoglobin concentration.

2. Relate anemia and its general symptoms to the physiological role of hemoglobin.

3. Understand the mechanism that maintains the number of red cells at a normal level, and describe when and where cells are produced and destroyed.

4. Describe the metabolism of iron, its reutilization in the body, and how its absorption, transfer, and storage are controlled.

5. Recognize that the normal red cell contains a small amount of hemoglobin A_2, and, during fetal life, hemoglobin F, and that these two hemoglobins can be produced to replace hemoglobin A, if there is a restricted capacity for its synthesis.

6. Describe the possible causes of anemia, including defects in protein structure and in the red cell.

7. Examine a blood sample to see if the red cells and hemoglobin are normal, and perform tests to diagnose the abnormality.

The article following this chapter describes investigations of properties of red cells in an hereditary disease called *spherocytosis*. In this paper the authors use a number of techniques which include the use of radioactive iron and chromium to study the survival of red cells in the patient before and after removal of the spleen. The implications of their findings merit discussion.

LABORATORY INVESTIGATION: EXPERIMENTAL ANEMIA

Inject under the skin of a rat, on four consecutive days, 2 ml of a freshly prepared and neutralized solution of 0.25% phenylhydrazine (this hemolyzes red cells). Investigate the recovery process every second day, using methods learned in Chapter 1. This should be done for two weeks. Prepare a report with your data and conclusions.

ANEMIA

Anemia is the clinical name for an abnormally low hemoglobin content in blood. It results in a shortage of oxygen transportation, and the more sensitive cells begin to suffer. Symptoms develop in the brain (headache and vertigo), heart (pain on exertion), muscle (weakness), and eventually even in the skin (loss of elasticity, glazed sore tongue, spoon-shaped nails). Heart speeds increase, and respiration becomes deep and more rapid in an attempt to compensate for the decrease of hemoglobin.

Red cells have a limited life span, usually around 120 days. To compensate for this, they are continually produced in the bone marrow. The process begins with an undifferentiated cell, which starts to accumulate iron and undergoes four cell divisions. During this stage the cell and its nucleus become smaller (*pyknotic*). The cytoplasm is full of ribosomes which synthesize hemoglobin, and this slowly accumulates. Then the ribosomes begin to disappear, and the nucleus is ejected from the cell. A cell without a nucleus and with some ribosomes is called a *reticulocyte*. In a day or two the reticulocyte moves into the bone marrow capillaries, where the last ribosomes are lost and the cell finally matures, taking the normal red cell shape. The whole process takes about five days.

As red cells get older and become incapable of replacing their protein, they become more fragile. Here the destruction process takes over and the spleen plays an important role. This organ is similar to a sponge and is filled with blood. The arteries that bring in the blood ramify, ending in small sac-like

RBC dia $\approx 7.8 - 8.6\mu$
$v\lambda \approx 80\mu^3$

structures called *splenic sinuses*. These sinuses have walls with pores of about 6μ. Connecting the pores and lying between sinuses are the *Bilroth cords*, which contain phagocytic cells. The blood entering the spleen flows through the cords, and the phagocytic cells engulf and destroy only the old red cells. The blood then flows back into the sinuses and from them to veins which lead out of the spleen. Red cells that cross the gap into the cords are submitted to low oxygen and glucose concentration, and, through a process not yet understood, are *conditioned* to be destroyed. Older or abnormal cells are the only ones conditioned by this passage in the spleen. They are then destroyed either in the spleen itself, in the liver, or in the bone marrow.

The number of red cells in the body depends on the rates of production and destruction. It has been shown that the blood plasma of animals made anemic by bleeding contains a special protein, which, when injected into other animals, induces increased production of red cells. This protein is called *erythropoietin*. It is produced by the kidneys from a plasma precursor when they receive too little oxygen. The kidneys supply an enzyme which breaks the precursor, releasing *entropoietin* (molecular weight 39,000). The same process occurs in humans moving to higher altitudes, where oxygen concentration is lower and more red cells are needed. This leads us to assume that entropoietin is the regulator of red cell production, and that it maintains a suitable number of cells even under changing circumstances.

One can envision anemia as being due to (1) *deficiency in red cell production* (which may be caused by a deficiency of nutrients such as iron and vitamins, a deficiency in the production of erythropoietin, or a lack of proerythroblasts in the bone marrow), (2) *increase in red cell destruction* (due either to defects in the red cells which shorten their lives or to an overactive destruction mechanism), or (3) *blood loss* (hemorrhages, intestinal worms, etc.)

In the laboratory experiment, anemia was produced in rats by a hemolysis-inducing drug. You may have observed an increase in rate and depth of respiration, as well as an increased heart rate resulting in a more efficient utilization of red cells. An incomplete saturation of red cells by oxygen results in an increased production of DPG, which changes the dissociation curve of hemoglobin, making possible a larger release of oxygen (see Chapter 2, Figures 2-20 and 2-21). But these mechanisms cannot overcome a severe anemia. The partial anoxia in the kidney results in the production of entropoietin. More undifferentiated bone marrow cells start to produce red cells. Reticulocytes, and even some cells which still have nuclei, are released into the bloodstream to replace the ones destroyed. The blood examinations in the experiment should have detected this.

A number of drugs, like antibiotics (chloramphenicol, penicillin, tetra-cyclines), anticonvulsants (trimethadione), analgesics (phenylbutazone), and chemicals (benzene and derivatives), as well as ionizing radiations, can interfere with the normal production of red cells in bone marrow, inducing a transitory or permanent *aplastic* anemia. The diagnosis of abnormal bone marrow is made by puncturing a bone (sternum or vertebra) and removing a tissue sample. The tissue is either smeared or cut and stained. The examination of bone marrow preparation is rather complex and requires identifying red cells in the several stages of differentiation, from the undifferentiated bone marrow cell to the reticulocyte, and distinguishing them from the various types of white cells that are also in process of differentiation.

Iron Deficiency Anemia

The normal iron content for an adult man is about 4 g, 66 percent being found in hemoglobin and 4 percent in myoglobin. The important iron proteins in the cell, related to cell respiration, represent less than 1 percent of the total content, while 29 percent is stored in reserve. Hemoglobin is therefore the most important iron-containing compound in the body, from the medical point of view. It clearly has the highest turnover of iron: three million red cells must be produced each second, and it requires 21 mg of iron to make the 6.3 g of hemoglobin produced each day.

Practically all the iron from the destroyed red cells is reutilized, and a man needs only 0.5 mg per day to compensate for losses in the feces or from skin shedding. If he received no iron in his diet and did not lose blood, it would take several years before he developed an iron-deficiency anemia. Women, due to menstrual losses, need 1 mg per day, and this need goes as high as 6 mg in the last half of pregnancy, when the fetus must be supplied with the iron it needs. This continues until the baby begins to receive iron from food other than its mother's milk.

Iron can be absorbed only in the reduced form (Fe^{++}). Part of the iron in the diet is reduced in the stomach by hydrochloric acid. Iron may also combine with compounds in the diet, such as ascorbic acid, and hence remain soluble. Other compounds, such as plant phytic acid, form insoluble salts with iron and render it nonabsorbable. Only 1 to 17 percent of the iron present in the diet is absorbed, and this changes according to the body's needs.

Iron is absorbed by the intestine and stored in the oxidized form (Fe^{+++}) in the intestinal wall. It is then transferred to blood plasma and attached to a protein called *transferrin.* This protein is essential in the transportation of iron to the bone marrow and liver, where it attaches to the membrane of the differentiating red cells, releasing iron into their cytoplasm. In some very rare patients who do not have transferrin, iron is distributed to other organs, where it is deposited in the cells in a form not useful for hemoglobin synthesis.

Iron is stored in cells, and later used, as part of a complex, *ferritin,* containing a specific protein, *apoferritin.* Ferritin is a molecule with a molecular weight of 480,000, made up of many identical protein subunits which surround a core containing eight atoms of iron that are present in the form of hydroxide and phosphate. The complex is large enough to be detected by electron microscopy. Part of the iron can form larger aggregates, having a higher iron concentration and appearing as granules, that properly stained can be seen under the light microscope. They are known as *hemosiderin* and constitute a storage form more stable than ferritin.

It has been suggested that when the reserves of iron are high, all apoferritin in the intestinal cells is in the form of ferritin, and this limits the absorption of iron from food.

Iron from ferritin is transferred to the mitochondria of the red cell precursor. There it combines with protoporphyrin to form heme. Heme in turn combines with globins in the cytoplasm to form hemoglobin. If there is a defect in the biosynthesis of protoporphyrin (as in lead poisoning), the mitochondria will remain charged with iron and burst. In the red cell precursors in the bone marrow this is detected as a ring surrounding the nucleus. In blood smear preparations it is evident from small granules in red cells. Both the ring and the granules stain as iron.

Iron deficiency develops when there is blood loss (acute blood loss or a more chronic condition, such as that caused by intestinal worms or abnormal menstruation), inadequate intestinal absorption (caused by lack of hydrochloric acid in the stomach secretion or by improper pancreatic secretion), or lack of transferrin. The hemoglobin level in the blood goes down, and red cells become smaller (microcytic with MVC smaller than 87) and paler (hypochromic, with MCHC smaller than 30).

Iron deficiency is the most common medical disorder, and is a major public health problem among poor people (especially women and children) and in developing countries. It can be corrected easily by an oral daily dose of 100 to 200 mg of iron (as ferrous sulphate). Parenteral iron is used only when a rapid response is necessary or when there is a gastrointestinal disorder that makes oral administration inadequate. It is frequently given as a red cell transfusion. An overdose of parenteral iron is very toxic and cannot be corrected easily. Even large oral overdoses of iron (that occur with children that ingest iron tablets) may result in shock, coma, and death.

Anemia from Other Deficiencies

Bone marrow cells are rapidly dividing cells and hence are very sensitive to some nutritional deficiencies — specifically, folic acid and vitamin B_{12}. These vitamins are essential in the synthesis of nucleic acids, which are required for cell division and protein synthesis. (The stomach produces a certain protein that is the intrinsic factor required for the absorption of vitamin B_{12}.) When they are not provided in the diet, or are not absorbed, large abnormal cells appear (MCV $>$ 10; MCHC = 31–35). This condition is called *pernicious* or *megaloblastic* anemia.

There are some very rare forms of anemia, correctable by pyridoxine in large doses, whose mechanism is yet unknown.

LABORATORY INVESTIGATION: DIAGNOSIS OF ANEMIAS

Obtain blood samples and clinical histories from patients suspected of being anemic. Investigate for abnormalities in the red cells, using the methods you already know and performing the following tests:

1. What happens to the shape of the red cells when the blood on a microscope slide is treated with a drop of fresh 2% sodium metabisulfide? (This converts all oxyhemoglobin to hemoglobin.)

2. At what concentration of sodium chloride do red cells begin to hemolyze, and how dilute should sodium chloride be to hemolyze all red cells?

3. If the hemoglobin spectrum is abnormal, compare it with the spectrum of a normal hemoglobin solution treated with a crystal of potassium ferricyanide. This converts all the hemoglobin (containing Fe^{++}) to methemoglobin (containing Fe^{+++}).

4. Test to see if the hemoglobin behaves normally (a) when treated with an alkaline solution, (b) when oxygen is removed, and (c) when migrating in an electric field (electrophoresis).

Osmotic Fragility of the Red Cell

Take twelve test tubes and label them 14 through 25. These numbers indicate the number of drops of 0.5% sodium chloride to be placed in each tube. Now add distilled water until there is a total of 25 drops in each tube. Mix thoroughly. You now have concentrations ranging from 0.28% to 0.50%. Add a drop of blood to each of the tubes, and mix. After two hours, centrifuge and see at what point the red cells begin to hemolyze and at what concentration hemolysis is complete.

Alkaline Resistance of Hemoglobin

Hemolyze red cells by adding 1.5 volumes of $1.15M$ NaOH and 0.5 volumes of toluene. Shake for 10 minutes and centrifuge for 20 minutes. Aspirate the two upper phases.

Add 0.8 ml of 0.1N NaOH to 0.1 ml of hemolyzate. After 60 seconds add 1.7 ml of ammonium sulfate (150 g ammonium sulfate in 200 ml of water and 10 ml of $1M$ HCl; dilute to 400 ml with distilled water). Keep in an ice bath for an hour, then centrifuge. Compare the color of the supernatant (which contains hemoglobin) with a hemolyzate diluted with water instead of with the other reagents.

Solubility of Hemoglobin

Take 0.2 ml of the hemolyzate prepared by the preceding method, and mix with 1.8 ml of a phosphate buffer ($1.62M$ K_3HPO_4 and $1.18M$ KH_2PO_4) and 25 mg of sodium hydrosulfite. After 15 minutes filter or centrifuge to remove any insoluble hemoglobin. Compare the color with a hemolyzate treated with water only.

Paper Electrophoresis

(Refer to Appendix II, Electrophoresis.)

Prepare a solution of barbiturate buffer pH 8.6, ionic strength 0.05 (sodium diethyl barbiturate 10.3 g, diethyl barbituric acid 0.9 g, and water to 1.0 liter).

Fill the electrode chambers of the apparatus and place paper strips (2.5 cm wide) running from one chamber to the other. Equalize the level of the buffer in the two chambers and let the paper strips equilibrate for 15 minutes with the chambers closed. With a micropipette, add 20 μl of hemolyzed red cells. Turn on the power, running the separation for 16 hours at 190 volts. (*Warning:* This DC voltage is very dangerous.) Disconnect the power supply. Remove the strips and dry them in an oven. Hemoglobin spots can be located by their color or by staining with benzidine-peroxide (0.5 ml acetic acid, 0.2 g benzidine, and 2 ml 3% hydrogen peroxide, diluted to 100 ml with water).

GLOBIN DEFECTS

Thalassemia

In 1925 Cooley described a severe form of anemia, present among people from the Mediterranean basin and the Orient (and their descendants who have migrated to other areas). It is known as *Cooley's anemia* or *thalassemia,* and results from an incapacity to produce one type of hemoglobin chain. Red cells are abnormally thin, and in stained preparations they may look like a bull's eye, with a central area of condensed hemoglobin surrounded by a clearer area. These are described as *target cells.*

When there is a block in the synthesis of beta chains, there may be an over-production of delta chains, increasing the proportion of hemoglobin A_2. There may also be production of fetal hemoglobin in the adult, to compensate for very severe anemia. This fetal hemoglobin is characterized by its alkaline resistance.

In another form of thalassemia, the block is in the production of alpha chains. In this case, part of the beta chains associate to form hemoglobin H, containing four alpha chains. Hemoglobin H precipitates in the red cell membrane and leads to hemolysis. If alpha chain production is completely blocked in a fetus, the fetus will produce only gamma chains (Barth's hemoglobin), which also associate to form a tetramer. This hemoglobin does not display the Bohr effect, and it leads to infant death by asphyxia.

Sickle Cell Anemia

Another type of abnormality, commonly found among Negroes and also among people in the Mediterranean region (and their descendants), is sickle cell anemia. When the red cells lose oxygen, hemoglobin molecules aggregate and precipitate like crystals. The cell is distorted, assuming a peculiar sickle-shaped form.* In 1949 Pauling showed that this hemoglobin has a different electrophoretic mobility from that of normal hemoglobin, and he proposed that sickle cell anemia was a molecular disease, i.e., a disease that results from a defect in molecular structure. In 1958 Ingram proved that Pauling's idea was correct, and the abnormality was shown to result from a substitution of a single valine for glutamic acid in the beta chains.

In the capillaries, when hemoglobin loses oxygen and is transformed into the sickle-shaped cells, viscosity increases, interfering with normal blood flow. Tissues remove more oxygen from the slow-flowing blood, causing more sickling. Depending on where this occurs in the body, there may be intense pain due to cell anoxia, with grave lesions to the organ.

Other Anemias

Today we know of about 100 different hemoglobins, all of which vary from the normal sequence by the placement of only a single amino acid. Some do not cause problems, since the hemoglobin remains functional. Others may change the hemoglobin oxygen affinity or the Bohr effect. Many are unstable, creating short-lived cells that must be replaced. The rapid destruction results

*Seen in the film by T. H. Ham and C. P. Emerson, *Sickling of Erythrocytes* (New York: Holt, Rinehart & Winston, Inc).

in deposits of iron and overproduction of compounds like urobilin which come from protoporphyrin. If production of red cells does not balance the destruction, anemia occurs.

The iron in hemoglobin is buried in a hydrophobic pocket and oxidizes to Fe^{+++} very slowly. Only traces of Fe^{+++} hemoglobin (*methemoglobin*) exist in normal blood. In some patients with abnormal globin due to amino acid substitution, the oxidation is rapid, and bluish methemoglobin, not capable of carrying oxygen, increases. These nonfunctional red cells are destroyed, thus having a very short life.

METABOLIC DEFECTS

Normal red cells have a mechanism which reduces any methemoglobin formed back to hemoglobin. However, a form of methemoglobinemia is found in which this reducing mechanism does not operate.

It has been known for many years that red cells can be preserved for transfusion for a longer period of time if glucose is added to the solution. Red cells are not in osmotic equilibrium with plasma, and must continuously excrete sodium and water, keeping up a high concentration of potassium. Glucose metabolism supplies the energy for this process and the reducing power to keep hemoglobin from being transformed into methemoglobin.

We know today that red cell destruction and anemia can result from defects of glucose metabolism in the red cells, and several types of such defects have been described. An important one is susceptibility to some drugs, specifically antimalarials. These seem to be capable of oxidizing hemoglobin, and when patients with defects in red cell glucose metabolism take them, massive hemolysis occurs, since the red cells cannot cope with the increasing need to reduce methemoglobin.

MEMBRANE DEFECTS

The red cell membrane is fundamental to maintaining the chemical constitution of the cell. It regulates not only the passive interchanges with the plasma but also the potassium and sodium levels, and it keeps the plasma slightly hypertonic. There are a few rare genetic diseases in which the red cell membrane is abnormal. It may also be abnormal in diseases involving abnormal lipid metabolism which brings about a chemical change in the lipids of the membrane. One rare disease is *hereditary spherocytosis,* in which small fragments break off from the red cell membrane. The membrane reseals, but to maintain the same volume the cell has to take a spherical shape because of the smaller surface area. In another strange disease, cells become susceptible to hemolysis when blood pH falls to 6.8 or lower. During sleep, when pulmonary ventilation is not efficient, the pH may go down and sudden hemolysis take place. This is called *paroxysmal nocturnal hemoglobinuria.* A sign of it is elimination of hemoglobin in urine.

To recognize these rare diseases, we must test the membrane's fragility. This can be done either by exposing the red cell to hypotonic concentrations and measuring the osmotic fragility, or by measuring membrane fragility during shaking or at low pH.

There is no method for correcting defects in the membrane or metabolism of red cells. Cells with this kind of abnormality have a very short life, which it is possible to lengthen by removing the spleen and thus eliminating conditioning for destruction. This avoids the stress of continuous overproduction of red cells and the toxic effects due to heme metabolism. It is known that the spleen also has some control over bone marrow, and removal of this organ causes the bone marrow to become more active in red cell production.

LABORATORY INVESTIGATION: BLOOD AND BONE MARROW SMEARS

1. Examine a collection of blood smears that include blood from (a) a normal person, (b) a patient who has recently had a hemorrhage, (c) a patient with iron deficiency anemia, (d) a patient with sickle cell anemia, and (e) a patient with vitamin B_{12} deficiency. Prepare a short report on each slide, giving the diagnosis and the reason for it.

2. Examine a bone marrow smear from a normal patient. Then examine two other slides. One is from a patient with severe aplastic anemia and the other from a patient who has had several hemorrhages. Try to identify them.

SELF-EVALUATION

1. The predominating hemoglobin in
   a. the fetus
   b. sickle cell anemia
   c. thalassemia
   d. hemolytic anemia

   has (choose one answer for each of the above)
   (p) normal alpha and beta chains.
   (q) beta chains with an amino acid substitution.
   (r) alpha chains with an amino acid substitution.
   (s) either no alpha or no beta chains.
   (t) two alpha and two delta chains.

2. a. Fetal hemoglobin
   b. Barth hemoglobin (four delta chains)
   c. S hemoglobin

   is characterized by (choose one answer for each of the above)
   (p) alkaline resistance.
   (q) insolubility of the hemoglobin form.
   (r) insolubility of the oxyhemoglobin.
   (s) absence of the Bohr effect.
   (t) being easily oxidized to methemoglobin.

3. The finding of
   a. target cells
   b. large red cells with nuclei
   c. sickle cells
   d. reticulocytosis

   strongly suggests (choose one for each of the above)
   (p) thalassemia.
   (q) a hemorrhage.
   (r) lack of vitamin B_{12}.
   (s) lack of folic acid.
   (t) hemolysis.
   (u) lack of iron.
   (v) a genetic disease.

4. A laboratory report of
   a. MCV 150 μ^3, MCHC 34 g/100 ml
   b. MCV 65 μ^3, MCHC 25 g/100 ml
   c. MCV 88 μ^3, MCHC 34 g/100 ml

   (choose one answer from each group for each report)

   is (p) microcytic, (q) macrocytic, (r) normocytic

   and (s) hypochromic, (t) hyperchromic, (u) normochromic

   and could be due to (v) hemorrhage, (w) hemolysis, (x) pernicious anemia,
   (y) iron deficiency, (z) sickle cell anemia.

5. The following is true of the relationship between kidney function and red
   cells:
   a. Iron is excreted in the urine.
   b. The kidney conditions red cells for destruction.
   c. The kidney can excrete the heme derivative after destruction of the red
      cells.
   d. The kidney is responsible for the activation of erythropoietin.

6. Iron combines with
   a. apoferritin
   b. transferrin
   c. globins

   (choose one or more answers for each of the above)
   (p) to form hemoglobin and myoglobin.
   (q) for storage.
   (r) for intestinal absorption.
   (s) for none of these.

ALTERATIONS IN OSMOTIC AND MECHANICAL FRAGILITY RELATED TO *IN VIVO* ERYTHROCYTE AGING AND SPLENIC SEQUESTRATION IN HEREDITARY SPHEROCYTOSIS*†

Robert C. Griggs‡, Russell Weisman, Jr., John W. Harris§

From the Department of Medicine, Western Reserve University School of Medicine at Cleveland Metropolitan General Hospital, and University Hospitals of Cleveland, Ohio. Submitted for publication July 20, 1959; accepted August 20, 1959

Increased osmotic and mechanical fragility of the erythrocytes is a consistent finding in patients with hereditary spherocytosis, although in a few individuals it is necessary to incubate the cells at 37°C. for 24 hours before the otherwise latent abnormality becomes demonstrable. Splenectomy will correct the hemolytic process of hereditary spherocytosis despite the continuing production of abnormally fragile cells by the patient. The spleen is, therefore, essential in the destruction of the intrinsically defective erythrocytes. In the peripheral blood of some individuals with this disease a "double population" of cells exists. One component consists of more markedly fragile cells that are not present after splenectomy and must, therefore, have been related to the presence of the spleen.

The present study was undertaken to investigate the changes in osmotic and mechanical fragility accompanying *in vivo* erythrocyte aging and splenic sequestration and to elucidate the source and fate of the more markedly fragile group of red cells found in some patients.

Advantage was taken of the increased erythropoiesis in patients with hereditary spherocytosis prior to splenectomy to label *in vivo* with Fe^{59} the new red cells produced during a short time span, thereby obtaining an identifiable group of cells of known age. Using techniques that will be described, it was possible to differentiate these isotopically-labeled cells from the other cells in the peripheral circulation and to compare their characteristics to those of the general population. The changes in osmotic and mechanical fragility occurring in these labeled red cells during *in vivo* aging and splenic sequestration were followed. In addition, erythrocytes were recovered from the spleen at the time of splenectomy and reinjected into the patient's peripheral circulation. The post-splenectomy survival and changes in osmotic and mechanical fragility of these cells, labeled with Cr^{51}, were followed and distinguished from the cells of the general population.

*A preliminary report of this work appeared in abstract form (J. Clin. Invest. 1958, 37, 899).
† This study was supported by a grant from the Webster-Underhill Fund and Public Health Service Grant No. A-745.
‡Webster-Underhill Fellow, Western Reserve University School of Medicine.
§ Markle Scholar in Medical Science, Western Reserve University School of Medicine

METHODS

Routine hematologic studies were performed by standard methods (1). Autohemolysis was determined by the method of Selwyn and Dacie (2) as modified by Young, Izzo, Altman and Swisher (3). Erythrocyte osmotic fragility tests were done as described by Emerson and associates (4) and the osmotic fragility of the labeled cells was distinguished from that of the general population by the following modification of this method. The volume of each saline solution was increased to 3 ml., and 0.3 ml. of defibrinated whole blood was added to each tube. These were then centrifuged, decanted and the hemoglobin content of 0.5 ml. of the supernatant solution determined in a Beckman (Model B) spectrophotometer. The remainder of the supernatant was transferred to a calibrated isotope counting tube and the radioactivity determined in a low background, well-type scintillation counter (Tracerlab). Sufficient counts were obtained to give a statistical error of ± 3 percent or less. As a blank, 0.3 ml. of the defibrinated whole blood was suspended in hypertonic saline (1.25 Gm. NaCl per 100 ml.) and the radioactivity found in this supernatant after centrifugation was subtracted from that obtained for the other samples. The value for radioactivity thus obtained represented isotope released by the red cells lysed at each concentration of sodium chloride. The amount of radioactivity in each sample was calculated as a percentage of that released into the supernatant when 0.3 ml. of the defibrinated whole blood had undergone complete hemolysis by addition to 3 ml. distilled water. The results were plotted as two curves, one showing the percentage of hemolysis measured as hemoglobin (the osmotic fragility of all the cells in the sample) and the other curve representing the percentage of radioactivity released at each concentration of sodium chloride (the osmotic fragility of only the isotopically labeled cells). Control studies demonstrated that no appreciable Fe^{59} was present in the stroma of the lysed cells and that osmotic fragility curves obtained by this isotope method on our patients after general distribution of the Fe^{59} through the red cell population were identical with those obtained by the usual method in which hemoglobin from lysed red cells is measured.

The mechanical fragility of the red cells was determined by a modification of the method of Shen, Castle and Fleming (5). The hematocrit of a sample of defibrinated venous blood was adjusted to 35 percent and 0.5 ml. subjected to the standardized trauma produced by rotating it for 90 minutes in a 50 ml. Erlenmeyer flask at 30 rpm with 10 uniform 4 mm. selected glass beads. To obtain an adequate sample for the isotope counting procedures, two flasks were used for each determination and combined after rotation. The results were corrected by a blank consisting of a similar blood sample in hypertonic saline (1.25 Gm. NaCl per 100 ml.) and expressed as percentage of hemolysis compared to hemolysis in distilled water.

Ten $\mu c.$ of Fe^{59} in the form of ferric chloride (Abbott) (3 to 10 $\mu g.$ of elemental iron) was incubated with 20 ml. of normal compatible heparinized plasma and administered intravenously to each patient. Since patients with hemolytic anemias have increased saturation of their iron-binding protein, normal compatible plasma was used instead of the patient's. The plasma Fe^{59} clearance and the red cell Fe^{59} utilization studies were performed according to the method of Huff and associates (6,7).

Red cell survival was determined by the method of Ebaugh, Emerson and Ross (8) using 120 μc. of Cr[51]. In each case the patient's own red cells, obtained from either peripheral vein or splenic pulp, were used. Intact red cells were recovered from the spleen at operation. Using sterile technique, this was accomplished by making a number of large incisions into the surgical specimen immediately after removal and allowing the formerly entrapped blood to flow into a glass flask where it was defibrinated by rotating with glass beads.

Scintillation counting over the body surface was done by the methods described by Huff and co-workers (7) and Jandl, Greenberg, Yonemoto and Castle (9). The counting rates over the liver and spleen are plotted as ratios relative to the couting rate over the precordium.

RESULTS

Three unrelated adults who were referred to this hospital for investigation of anemia or jaundice were studied. All had splenomegaly and showed spherocytosis on peripheral blood smears; appropriate laboratory tests confirmed the diagnosis of hereditary spherocytosis. Family history in all three was negative for anemia, jaundice or splenomegaly. The mother of Case 2 was the only relative available for examination and her blood studies, including osmotic and mechanical fragility, were normal. Identifying data and laboratory findings are recorded in Table I. Presplenectomy studies with Fe[59] were performed on Cases 1 and 2 and post-splenectomy studies with Cr[51] on Cases 2 and 3.

Presplenectomy Studies

Case 1 showed evidence of a marked hemolytic process. A Cr[51] autosurvival had been performed in our laboratory on this individual one year prior to the present study and demonstrated a red cell half-life of eight days compared to a normal of at least 28 days for this method. During the present study he showed a marked hyperbilirubinemia (indirect reacting) and sustained reticulocytosis (Table I). Both the spleen and liver were enlarged. The administered Fe[59] was rapidly cleared from the plasma, with a half-time of 15 minutes contrasted to a normal of 60 to 120 minutes. The utilization of Fe[59] for red cell formation and the distribution of body surface counts are represented in Figure 1. There was rapid incorporation of Fe[59] into new red cells as might be anticipated in a patient with hemolytic anemia. This reached a maximum of 65 percent on Day 6. Body surface counting demonstrated early and rapid accumulation of isotope in the spleen after the expected initial rise and fall in counting rate over the sacral bone marrow.

Peripheral blood samples were studied at frequent intervals for changes in erythrocyte fragility by the osmotic and mechanical fragility methods described above. There was not sufficient radioactivity present in the red cells prior to the third day to give statistically valid counting rates. The results of the studies of the osmotic fragility on Days 3, 7, 10, 13, 24 and 30 are presented in Figure 2. The osmotic fragility of the patient's total peripheral red cell population is increased. The lower portion of the fragility curve shows some asymmetry with approximately 20 percent of the cells being more markedly fragile than the other red cells in the peripheral blood. The broken lines represent the osmotic fragility of the Fe[59]-labeled red cells. Since the labeling of the

Table 1. Laboratory data on patients in study

Case	Age Race Sex	Hgb.* Gm.%	Hct. %	Retics. %	Bilirubin direct total mg./100 ml.		Erythrocyte osmotic fragility	Erythrocyte mechanical fragility 0 hrs. % 1–5	24 hrs. % 9–15	% Autohemolysis 48 hours No glucose	With glucose	Plasma clearance Fe59 half-time min.	Erythrocyte survival Cr51 half-time days
Normal range										0–3	0–1	60–120	28+
1	68 W M	10	30	15	1.4	5.1	Increased	22	37	12.4	8.3	15	8
2	32 N F	9.5	32	4	0.7	1.1	Increased	18	37			31	
3	54 W M	9.5	29	3	0.5	1.0	Increased	7	17	5.7	1.5		16

*Hgb. = hemoglobin: Hct. = hematocirt: Retics. = reticulocytes.

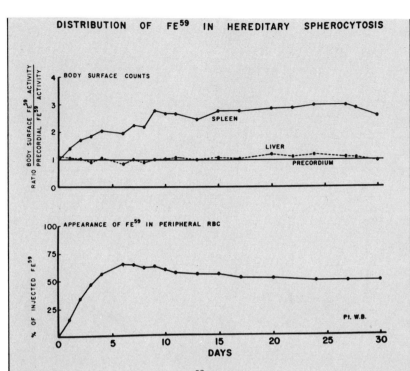

Fig. 1. Case 1: Utilization of Fe^{59} for red cell formation and *in vivo* distribution.

red cells is occurring as they are formed *in vivo*, on Day 3 all cells represented by this curve must be no more than three days old. The fragility curves of these new cells on Days 3 and 7 show some increase in fragility as compared to normal red cells, but do not have the asymmetrical curve of the total peripheral cell population and none of the cells are as osmotically fragile as some of the red cells in the peripheral blood. It is not until Day 10 and subsequently that some of the labeled cells show fragility changes comparable to that of the general cell population.

During the early phases of this study, observations were also made on cells after sterile incubation for 24 hours. However, no difference was noted between the fragility of the labeled cells and the general peripheral population, and these studies were not continued. All observations reported are on fresh, unincubated whole blood.

The concurrent changes in mechanical fragility of red cells of Case 1 are depicted on the lower half of Figure 3. The mechanical fragility of this patient's peripheral red cells varied from 18 to 27 percent compared to a normal of 1 to 3 percent by this method. On Day 3 the mechanical fragility of the new red cells as measured by the Fe^{59} was 10 percent. This gradually increased until it was equal to that of the total cell population (24 percent) on Day 13. Subsequently, the labeled cells exhibited a mechanical fragility slightly increased above that of the general population.

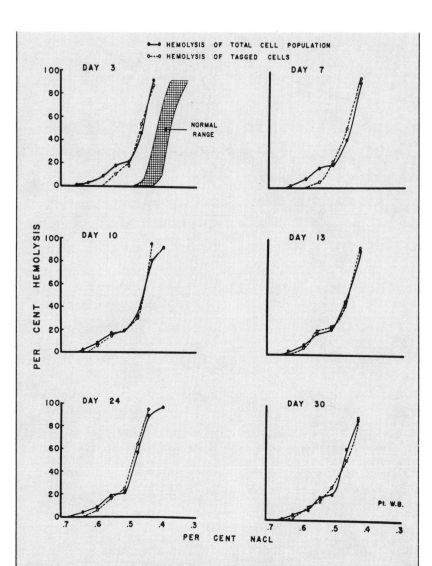

Fig. 2. Case 1: Osmotic fragility of the Fe^{59}-labeled red cells contrasted with that of the total peripheral cell population.

A similar study was performed on Case 2 and the results are outlined in Figures 3 through 5. This individual showed evidence of a less severe hemolytic process, a reticulocytosis of 4 percent and no hyperbilirubinemia (Table 1). The half-time for plasma clearance of Fe^{59} was 31 minutes with rapid reappearance of the isotope in the peripheral red cells. This reached a maximum recorded utilization of 80 percent on Day 10. There was evidence by body surface counting of gradual accumulation of Fe^{59} in the spleen (Figure 4). Studies of osmotic fragility

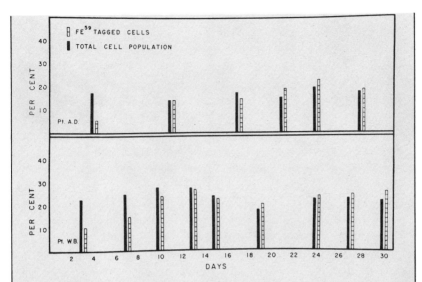

Fig. 3. Mechanical fragility of the Fe59-labeled cells contrasted with that of the total peripheral cell population in Cases 1 (W.B.) and 2 (A.D.).

similar to those described above were performed on this patient and the results are presented in Figure 5. In an effort to diminish the reutilization of Fe59 from destroyed red cells in further red cell production, a relatively large dose of nonisotopic iron was administered beginning on Day 11 of the study. From Day 11 to Day 28, 950 mg. of iron was administered in divided doses intramuscularly in the form of Imferon®. Approximately 15 percent of this patient's peripheral red cells showed a marked increase in osmotic fragility as represented by the lower portion of the curve (solid lines, Figure 5). On Day 4 the new Fe59-labeled red cells, represented by the broken line, did not show any cells with this marked increase in fragility. By Day 11 the proportion of fragile cells had increased and by Day 17 the proportion had increased above that of the general peripheral cell population and about 20 percent of the cells showed a marked increase in fragility. These very fragile cells then apparently disappeared from the peripheral circulation within several days, for the fragility curve of the labeled cells on Day 24 is similar to that seen on Day 4. Subsequent studies, not shown in the figures, demonstrated that a portion of the labeled cells again became more fragile and both curves were essentially the same after Day 31.

The results of the mechanical fragility studies on this patient are presented in the upper half of Figure 3. As in the previous study, the mechanical fragility of the labeled cells was initially low and then gradually increased, eventually becoming slightly greater than that of the general cell population.

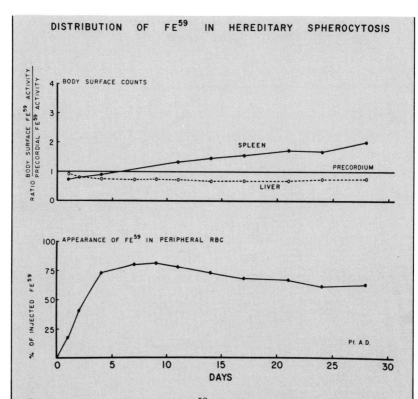

Fig. 4. Case 2: Utilization of Fe^{59} for red cell formation and *in vivo* distribution.

Splenectomy and Post-Splenectomy Studies

Cases 2 and 3 were studied during and after elective splenectomy for correction of the hemolytic process. In Case 2, intact red cells were recovered from the splenic pulp at the time of splenectomy. The osmotic fragility of these cells is shown in the upper left hand graph of Figure 6. As described previously by Emerson and associates (4), these cells were considerably more osmotically fragile than those found in the peripheral blood represented by the solid lines in Figure 5. Approximately 25 percent of the cells showed a marked increase in fragility. These spleen-drip cells were labeled with Cr^{51} and at the conclusion of the operative procedure, reinjected into a peripheral vein after suitable filtration. Differential osmotic and mechanical fragility studies of a small sample of these cells indicated that the curve for Cr^{51} release on hemolysis of the cells was identical with the curve for hemoglobin liberation. The studies of Gray and Sterling (10) showed that 95 percent of the red cell Cr^{51} was bound to the hemoglobin; Necheles, Weinstein and Leroy (11) found only 78 percent with the hemoglobin fraction.

Starting one hour after reinjection peripheral blood samples were taken at frequent intervals. The survival of the chromium-labeled cells

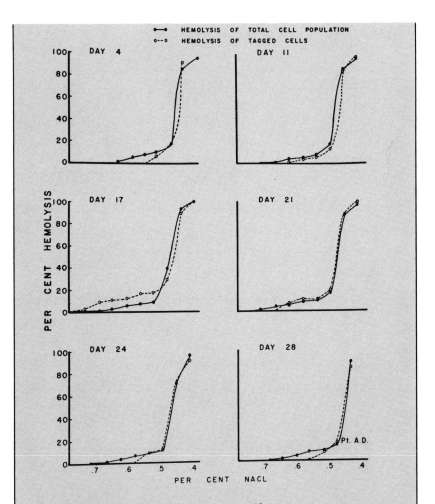

Fig. 5. Case 2: Osmotic fragility of the Fe[59]-labeled red cells contrasted with that of the total peripheral cell population.

was followed and, in addition, the changes in osmotic and mechanical fragilities of the labeled cells were studied in a manner similar to that used for the Fe[59]-labeled cells in the previous experiments. These results are presented in Figures 6 through 8. In Figure 6 the changes in osmotic fragility are recorded. The broken lines represent the isotope-labeled, spleen-drip cells and the solid lines represent the osmotic fragility of the peripheral cell population. Even one hour after reinjection of the labeled cells, there has been some change in the osmotic curve with a decrease in the number of markedly fragile cells. In the subsequent seven days there were further decreases in the fragile cells, until by Day 7 the two curves were essentially the same. There also has been a decrease in the number of markedly fragile cells in the

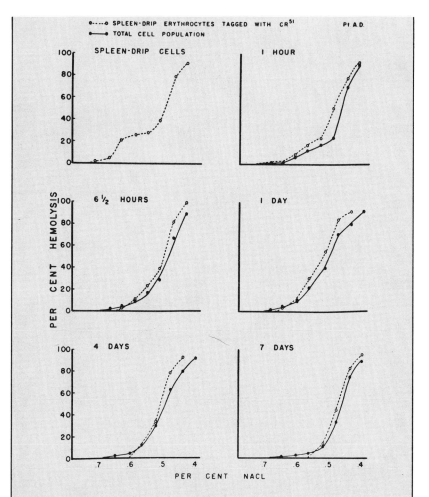

Fig. 6. Case 2: Changes in osmotic fragility of spleen-drip red cells labeled with Cr^{51} and retransfused into the patient post-splenectomy contrasted with the osmotic fragility of the total peripheral red cell population.

peripheral blood as a whole, so that the curve of hemolysis has become more symmetrical than before splenectomy.

The concurrent changes in mechanical fragility are seen in Figure 7. Twenty-seven percent of the spleen-drip cells and 20 percent of the peripheral cells were destroyed by the standard trauma. Both gradually showed less marked fragility, the labeled cells showing a more rapid change, both mechanical fragilities being essentially the same by Day 13.

The survival of these Cr^{51}-labeled, spleen-drip red cells is presented in Figure 8. The one hour postinjection sample, the first one obtained, was plotted as 100 percent. During the first 48 hours there was a rapid

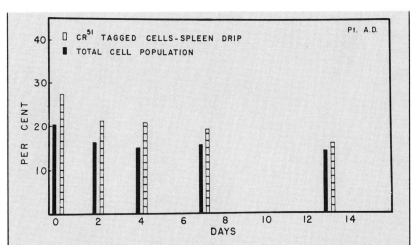

Fig. 7. Case 2: Changes in mechanical fragility of spleen-drip red cells labeled with Cr[51] and retransfused into the patient post-splenectomy contrasted with the mechanical fragility of the total peripheral red cell population.

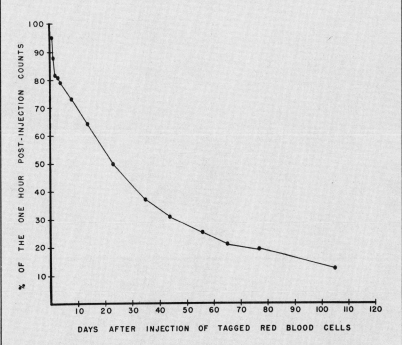

Fig. 8. Case 2: Survival of spleen-drip red cells labeled with Cr[51] and retransfused into the patient post-splenectomy. (Data are not corrected for chromium elution.)

loss of approximately 20 percent of the labeled cells. The remainder of
the cells showed a normal length of survival.

A similar study of the postsplenectomy survival of spleen-drip red
cells was performed on Case 3 and the findings recorded in Figure 9.
The solid line represents the Cr^{51} autosurvival of this patients' red cells
done in our laboratory several months prior to splenectomy. A half-life
of 16 days was obtained. A sample of cells obtained from the spleen at
the time of splenectomy was labeled with Cr^{51} and reinjected into the
peripheral circulation postoperatively. About 30 percent of these cells
showed a marked increase in osmotic fragility. The survival curve
(broken line, Figure 9) reveals that 50 percent of the autotransfused red
cells were removed from the circulation within 48 hours; the remaining
cells had a normal life span of 100 to 120 days. Neither of these patients
showed any significant blood loss postoperatively and on follow-up
studies over a period of months, both patients have shown the anticipated good clinical response.

DISCUSSION

The clinical picture and pathologic physiology of hereditary spherocytosis have been reviewed recently in some detail by Dacie (12) and
Young (13). Only a brief outline will be presented here of the erythrocyte

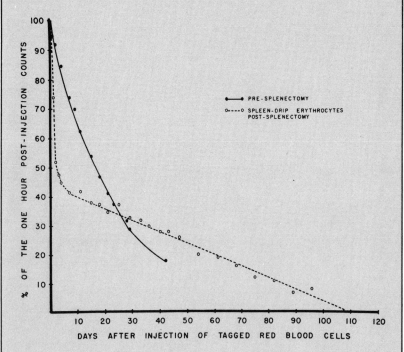

Fig. 9. Case 3: Survival of spleen-drip red cells labeled with Cr^{51} and
retransfused into the patient post-splenectomy. (Data are not corrected
for chromium elution.)

abnormalities and of the role of the spleen in the hemolytic process. The relationship of these two factors, the abnormal red cell and the spleen, has been most concisely demonstrated in a study of red cell survival by Emerson (14). He showed that normal red cells had a normal survival in a patient with hereditary spherocytosis, but that the patient's red cells were incapable of normal survival in a recipient *except* in the absence of a spleen. Although patients with hereditary spherocytosis characteristically have an enlarged spleen, there is no primary abnormality of the spleen, since it has been amply demonstrated both *in vivo* and *in vitro* that a spleen from a patient with hereditary spherocytosis and one from a normal individual will both selectively remove perfused spherocytic red cells but will not selectively remove normal red cells. Although maturing erythrocytes in the patient's bone marrow may show some minor shape changes, they evidently become more abnormal in shape shortly after release into the peripheral circulation (12). Abnormalities in glucose and phosphate metabolism have been demonstrated in these cells (15), but probably related to the abnormal thickness of the cells and their inability to escape easily through slit-like openings in the venous sinusoids (12), the spheroidal cells are trapped in the spleen. The entrapped cells are evidently in a deleterious environment, which perhaps, in combination with the deficiencies of metabolism that these spherocytes demonstrate, eventually results in alterations in the cells. These changes have been designated by the term "conditioning," and are recognized by abnormally increased osmotic and mechanical fragility. These "conditioned" cells may then either be destroyed in the spleen as evidenced by the elevated bilirubin level in splenic vein blood (12), or, escaping into the peripheral circulation, be identified as the markedly fragile portion of the osmotic curve. These markedly fragile cells are not found in the peripheral circulation of all individuals with hereditary spherocytosis, but their relationship to the spleen has been well established by the experiments of Young, Platzer, Ervin and Izzo (16). Dacie (12), Emerson and associates (4), and Weisman, Ham, Hinz and Harris (17), who have shown that fragile cells of this type are found in the spleen pulp and they are not present in the peripheral blood of patients after splenectomy.

In the present study an identifiable group of spherocytic red cells was produced in patients with hereditary spherocytosis by *in vivo* labeling with Fe^{59}. It is well established that iron administered in this fashion is incorporated only into new red cells and not into older cells. However, when the red cell containing Fe^{59} is destroyed, the iron is reutilized for new cell production. In an individual with normal red cell survival and normal iron metabolism, no reutilization would occur for 100 to 120 days. Red cells were rapidly being destroyed in the patients in the present study so that Fe^{59} was, to some degree, being incorporated repeatedly into new cells. This fact limits the usefulness of this technique for studying the cells for a prolonged period of time. Despite this objection it was possible to demonstrate progressive and significant changes in fragility of the new red cells and to follow them for approximately 30 days. Estimation of Fe^{59} incorporation into peripheral red cells by the usual techniques indicated a utilization of 65 percent in Case 1 and 80 percent in Case 2. This undoubtedly does not represent the true maximum utilization of the isotope for hemoglobin labeling since red cells containing Fe[59] were being continuously sequestered in in the spleen and therefore, removed from the peripheral circulation.

The osmotic fragility of the new red cells was found to be similar to the fragility of the majority of the cells in the peripheral blood. Of particular interest is the fact that none of the new erythrocytes was as osmotically fragile as some of the "conditioned" cells in the patient's peripheral blood. Thus, it is possible from this study to get some idea of the time required for the conditioning process. This would appear to be at least 10 days. From the present evidence it is impossible to say whether the cells are trapped in the spleen for the full period or the conditioning process is the result of recirculation or repeated short episodes of stagnation in the spleen.

Other investigators have studied the changes in red cell fragilities of dogs and humans without hematologic disease. Cruz, Hahn, Bale and Balfour (18), and later, Stewart, Stewart, Izzo and Young (19) using dog erythrocytes labeled *in vivo* with radioactive iron, found that newly formed cells were more osmotically fragile and less mechanically fragile than older cells. As they aged, they became more mechanically fragile, but the osmotic fragility was not significantly altered. In contrast, recent studies in normal man by Simon and Topper (20) and Marks and Johnson (21) have shown that normal young erythrocytes are more resistant to osmotic lysis than older cells.

The observations made after splenectomy on the survival and changes in osmotic and mechanical fragility of the spleen-drip red cells demonstrate that cells with the most marked abnormalities have a short survival and disappear from the circulation within 48 hours. The curves for osmotic fragility changes found in the spleen-drip red cells presented in Figure 6 suggest that there may have been some decrease in osmotic fragility between the time of reinjection of the labeled blood and the first sample studied one hour later. However, it seems more likely that some of the most fragile cells have already been eliminated from the peripheral circulation. Motulsky and co-workers (22) have suggested that the marked increase in osmotic fragility may revert toward normal if the cells are placed in a circulation without a spleen. He transfused red cells labeled with Cr[51] from a patient with hereditary spherocytosis, who had not undergone splenectomy and had a cell population consisting of approximately 30 percent very fragile cells, to the patient's splenectomized brother whose peripheral blood had no very fragile cells. The labeled donor cells showed a gradual decrease in osmotic fragility over a six day period. Since information on survival of these transfused cells is not presented, the observed changes could be due either to a reversible process in the very fragile red cells or to destruction and removal of these cells from the circulation. There is the possibility that the spleen-drip red cells studied in the present experiments had irreversible changes in contrast to the peripheral blood cells studied by Motulsky. He also performed the reverse experiment and transfused labeled red cells from the patient without a spleen into the brother with a spleen. Approximately six days were required for these red cells to show the marked increase in fragility seen in the recipient's own cell population.

The data from the present study demonstrate that in some patients with hereditary spherocytosis there is a progressive increase in osmotic and mechanical fragility of a portion of the red cell population, and that a period of approximately 10 days is required for these changes to reach their maximum from the time the cell first appears in the peripheral circulation. Previous information and the present study certainly implicate the spleen as the source of these very fragile red cells, since they can be found in the splenic pulp and are no longer seen in the peripheral blood after removal of the spleen. From information available at the present time it is impossible to say just how these red cells are conditioned in the spleen. Our experiments on the survival of red cells obtained from the spleen indicate that these very fragile cells have a short life span in the peripheral circulation, less than 48 hours. There was no evidence that the osmotic fragility of these cells reverted toward normal in the absence of the spleen. Therefore, it seems likely that in some patients with hereditary spherocytosis a significant proportion of the red cells is conditioned in the spleen over a period of days and escapes into the peripheral circulation, there undergoing rapid destruction either by the forces of mechanical trauma, osmotic lysis, or undertermined mechanisms.

SUMMARY

Changes in erythrocyte osmotic and mechanical fragility associated with aging and splenic sequestration were studied in two patients with hereditary spherocytosis by the use of Fe^{59}. New red cells showed some increase in fragility, but after approximately 10 days, conditioned cells with a marked increase in osmotic and mechanical fragility appeared in the peripheral circulation. At the time of splenectomy, red cells were recovered from the spleen, labeled with Cr^{51} and reinjected into the patient's peripheral circulation. The conditioned, most fragile cells disappeared rapidly, surviving less than two days; the other red cells, less osmotically and mechanically fragile, had a normal length of survival.

REFERENCES
1. Ham, T. H. A Syllabus of Laboratory Examinations in Clinical Diagnosis. Cambridge, Mass., Harvard University Press, 1950.
2. Selwyn, J. G., and Dacie, J. V. Autohemolysis and other changes resulting from the incubation in vitro of red cells from patients with congenital hemolytic anemia. Blood 1954, 9, 414.
3. Young, L. E., Izzo, M. J., Altman, K. I., and Swisher, S. N. Studies on spontaneous in vitro autohemolysis in hemolytic disorders. Blood 1956, 11, 977.
4. Emerson, C. P., Jr., Shen, S. C., Ham, T. H., Fleming, E. M., and Castle, W. B. Studies on the destruction of red blood cells. IX. Quantitative methods for determining the osmotic and mechanical fragility of red cells in the peripheral blood and splenic pulp; the mechanism of increased hemolysis in hereditary spherocytosis (congenital hemolytic jaundice) as related to the functions of the spleen. A.M.A. Arch. Intern. Med. 1956, 97, 1.
5. Shen, S. C., Castle, W. B., and Fleming, E. M. Experimental and clinical observations on increased mechanical fragility of erythrocytes. Science 1944, 100, 387.
6. Huff, R. L., Hennessy, T. G., Austin, R. E., Garcia, J. F., Roberts, B. M., and Lawrence, J. H. Plasma and red cell iron turnover in normal subjects and in patients having various hematopoietic disorders. J. Clin. Invest. 1950, 29, 1041.

7. Huff, R. L., Elmlinger, P. J., Garcia, J. F., Oda, J. M., Cockrell, M. C., and Lawrence, J. H. Ferrokinetics in normal persons and in patients having various erythropoietic disorders. J. Clin. Invest. 1951, 30, 1512.

8. Ebaugh, F. G., Jr., Emerson, C. P., and Ross, J. F. The use of radioactive chromium 51 as an erythrocyte tagging agent for determination of red cell survival in vivo. J. Clin. Invest. 1953, 32, 1260.

9. Jandl, J. H., Greenberg, M. S., Yonemoto, R. H., and Castle, W. B. Clinical determination of the sites of red cell sequestration in hemolytic anemias. J. Clin. Invest. 1956, 35, 842.

10. Gray, S. J., and Sterling, K. The tagging of red cells and plasma proteins with radioactive chromium. J. Clin. Invest. 1950, 29, 1604.

11. Necheles, T. F., Weinstein, I. M., and Leroy, G. V. Radioactive sodium chromate for the study of survival of red blood cells. I. The effect of radioactive sodium chromate on red cells. J. Lab Clin. Med. 1953, 42, 358.

12. Dacie, J. V. The Haemolytic Anaemias: Congenital and Acquired. New York, Grune and Stratton, 1954.

13. Young, L. E. Hereditary spherocytosis. Amer. J. Med. 1955, 18, 486.

14. Emerson, C. P. The influence of the spleen on the osmotic behavior and the longevity of red cells in hereditary spherocytosis (congenital hemolytic jaundice), a case study. Boston Med. Quart. 1954, 5, 65.

15. Prankerd, T. A. J., Altman, K. I., and Young, L. E. Abnormalities of carbohydrate metabolism of red cells in hereditary spherocytosis (abstract). J. Clin. Invest. 1954, 33, 957.

16. Young, L. E., Platzer, R. F., Ervin, D. M., and Izzo, M. J. Hereditary spherocytosis. II. Observations on the role of the spleen. Blood 1951, 6, 1099.

17. Weisman, R., Jr., Ham, T. H., Hinz, C. F., Jr., and Harris, J. W. Studies of the role of the spleen in the destruction of erythrocytes. Trans. Ass. Amer. Phycns 1955, 68, 131.

18. Cruz, W. O., Hahn, P. F., Bale, W. F., and Balfour, W. M. The effect of age on the susceptibility of the erythrocyte to hypotonic salt solutions. Radioactive iron as a means of tagging the red blood cell. Amer. J. Med. Sci. 1941, 202, 157.

19. Stewart, W. B., Stewart, J. M., Izzo, M. J., and Young, L. E. Age as affecting the osmotic and mechanical fragility of dog erythrocytes tagged with radioactive iron. J. Exp. Med. 1950, 91, 147.

20. Simon, E. R., and Topper, Y. J. Fractionation of human erythrocytes on the basis of their age. Nature (Lond.) 1957, 180, 1211.

21. Marks, P. A., and Johnson, A. B. Relationship between the age of human erythrocytes and their osmotic resistance: A basis for separating young and old erythrocytes. J. Clin. Invest. 1958, 37, 1542.

22. Motulsky, A. G., Casserd, F., Giblett, E. R., Broun, G. O., Jr., and Finch, C. A. Anemia and the spleen. New Eng. J. Med. 1958, 259, 1215.

FURTHER READINGS

Beck, W. S. (Ed.) *Hematology*. Cambridge, Mass.: M.I.T. Press, 1973.

Gordon, A. S. (Ed.) *Regulation of Hematopoiesis*. New York: Appleton-Century-Crofts, 1970.

Harris, J. K., and Kellermeyer, R. W. *The Red Cell*. Cambridge, Mass.: Harvard University Press, 1969.

Hyun, B. H., Blank, M., and Custer, R. C. *Hematology: A Filmstrip Presentation*. Philadelphia: Saunders, 1970.

Morimoto, H., Lehman, H., and Perutz, M. F. Molecular pathology of human hemoglobin: Stereochemical interpretation of abnormal oxygen affinities. *Nature* (Lond.) 232:408, 1971.

Perutz, M. F., and Lehman, H. Molecular pathology of human hemoglobin. *Nature* (Lond.) 219:902, 1968.

Stambury, J. B., Wyngaarden, J. B., and Fredrickson, D. S. *The Metabolic Basis of Inherited Diseases* (3rd ed.) New York: McGraw-Hill, 1972.

Williams, W., Beutler, E., Ersler, A., and Rundles, R. W. *Hematology*. New York: McGraw-Hill, 1972.

Zuckerkandl, E. and Pauling, L. Molecular Disease, Evolution and Genetic Heterogeneity. In Kasha, A., and Pullman, B., *Horizons in Chemistry*. New York: Academic, 1962.

4 From Molecules to Genetics

STUDY GUIDE

In the course of this unit you will be expected to do the following:

1. Apply Mendel's laws to data collected from a large number of families in order to establish the principles of inheritance of human characteristics. Use the chi-square method (Appendix VI) to calculate the probability of your interpretation's being correct.

2. Use Mendel's laws to provide genetic diagnosis for some common hereditary diseases, simple as well as sex-linked.

3. Study pedigrees, and deduce possible inheritance mechanisms for such traits based both on Mendel's laws and on linkage and crossing-over.

4. Discuss the scientific basis and some of the implications of genetic counseling.

MENDEL'S LAWS

When Mendel crossed pure round peas with a strain of pure wrinkled peas, he got a generation of round peas that on self-crossing gave three round to each wrinkled pea (Fig. 4-1). He correctly interpreted these results as being due to hypothetical hereditary factors, which today are known as *genes*. These genes are transmitted from generation to generation. For each trait, an individual has two genes, one from each parent. The pure strains for a specific characteristic have two of the same genes. Hybrids (known as *heterozygotes*) have two different genes for the same trait (two different *alleles*). One is *dominant* and

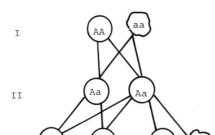

Fig. 4-1. Crossing of round and wrinkled peas.

expresses itself, and the other is *recessive.* The recessive gene is not destroyed but remains available for transmittance to descendants. Due to dominance, the apparent trait *(phenotype)* does not tell us about all the genes present *(genotype).*

Mendel then investigated two different traits at the same time: he studied round-yellow peas and wrinkled-green peas. In separate experiments he found that round and yellow were dominant. On cross-breeding he obtained, in the first generation, only round-yellow peas. In the second generation he obtained, as he had expected, a random assortment of combinations of color and texture: round-yellow, wrinkled-yellow, round-green and wrinkled-green, in the proportion 9:3:ɔ:1, thus 3:1 for round-wrinkled traits appeared in a proportion of 3:1, and yellow-green traits in a preparation of 3:1, showing that the genes for color and shape assorted independently.

LABORATORY INVESTIGATION: HEREDITARY TRAITS

1. Prepare a 0.1% solution of phenyl thicarbamide (PTC). Take about 2 ml in a spoon and see if you can taste it.

2. Can you roll your tongue upward at the sides?

3. Test a family for these two characteristics. Using your results, build a pedigree for the family, following Figure 4-2 as a model. When studying more than one trait at a time, make appropriate notations inside the symbols instead of simply darkening them.

4. Are the traits you studied hereditary? Can you explain them by using Mendel's laws?

Note: The concentration recommended for PTC is good enough for separating the people who taste from the people who do not taste, in 98 percent of the cases. Only about 2 percent of the tasters require stronger concentrations.

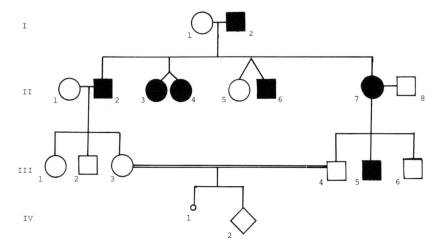

Fig. 4-2. Key to family pedigrees. Females are represented by circles, and males by squares. In generation II, 3 and 4 are identical twins, and 5 and 6 are fraternal twins. 1 and 2 are married, and 7 and 8 married. In generation III, 3 and 4, who are cousins, are married and have one child of unidentified sex (2) and a miscarriage (1). Double lines represent consanguineous marriages. Darkened signs identify the trait under study.

DOMINANCE

In Chapter 3, three criteria were given for sickle cell anemia: (1) the painful episodes that characterize the very sick patients; (2) the sickling phenomenon that occurs when red cells are made anaerobic; and (3) the presence of sickle cell anemia type hemoglobin.

A study of a family with sickle cell anemia gave the pedigree shown in Figure 4-3. A physician, through clinical examination, would detect those family members who have severe anemia and painful episodes (marked on the pedigree by fully shaded signs.) Affected children may have apparently normal parents. This would suggest a recessive gene. If laboratory tests for sickling are used, those family members with half-shaded signs will give positive results; that is, the abnormal gene will appear to be dominant in relation to the normal gene. A biochemist, on the other hand, would run electrophoretic tests to detect the different hemoglobins. Those family members marked with half-shaded signs would be found to have both normal and sickle cell hemoglobin, whereas those with a fully shaded sign, just sickle cell hemoglobin. He would

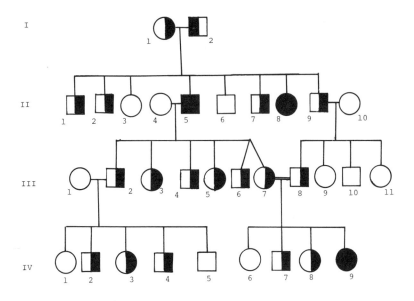

Fig. 4-3. Hypothetical pedigree of a family with a sickle cell trait.

be able to state then that there is no dominance (a situation sometimes called *codominance*).

In the case of sickle cell anemia, we know that the result of the gene action is expressed in hemoglobin. In the heterozygote, both the normal and the sickle cell genes are active, and a mixture of the two hemoglobins will be present. It is only when no A_1 (normal) hemoglobin is produced that the symptoms will be pronounced and will produce anemia. In another disease — thalassemia — the abnormality is that there is one inactive gene; that is, a hemoglobin chain is not produced. Therefore in the heterozygous condition, the hemoglobin produced is normal. In the homozygous condition one hemoglobin chain (alpha or beta) is not produced. For a large number of other hereditary traits like tasting PTC we do not know the first genetically induced biochemical product in the sequence of reactions that leads to the phenotype. We can only observe the symptoms and determine whether the abnormal gene seems dominant or recessive.

The phenomenon of dominance is not completely understood. In some hereditary diseases the expression appears to be variable: some patients are more affected than others. In other diseases, symptoms may appear late in life, suggesting the possibility of changes in dominance. It is known that changing conditions (in plants and animals) can change dominance.

RATIOS

In a marriage AA × AS, where A stands for a normal hemoglobin gene and S for a sickle cell gene, the ideal ratio of affected to unaffected children is 1:1, half the children possessing the AS genotype and the other half possessing AA (See Figure 4-4). This ratio does not tell us anything about a specific child. If such a family already has three AS children, the next one still has a 50 percent chance of being AS. The probabilities are unchanged by repetition (as in the case of flipping a coin).

Fig. 4-4. Expected ratio of offspring of an AA × AS couple.

		AS	
		A	S
AA	A	AA	AS
	A	AA	AS

As the number of children may be too small, frequently one does not find an ideal 1:1 ratio. In a family of four children from a marriage AA × AS, the various possibilities are as follows:

AA AA AA AA   4AA   AS AS AS AS   4AS

AA AA AA AS ⎫   AA AA AS AS ⎫
AA AA AS AA ⎬ 3AA:1AS   AA AS AA AS ⎪
AA AS AA AA ⎭   AA AS AS AA ⎬ 2AA:2AS
AS AA AA AA   AS AA AA AS ⎪
                                  AS AA AS AA ⎪
AS AS AS AA ⎫   AS AS AA AA ⎭
AS AS AA AS ⎬ 3AS:1AA
AS AA AS AS ⎪
AA AS AS AS ⎭

Only 6 out of 16 families of four children have the ideal 1:1 ratio.

In a marriage AS × AS the ideal ratio is 1SS: 2AS: 1AA. Using the same line of reasoning as before, we can calculate the probable number of families for each combination of children (parentheses indicate number of children having at least one sickle cell gene):

4SS	1	⎫		3SS: 1AA	4	⎫	
3SS: 1AS	8	⎬		2SS: 1AS: 1AA	24	⎬	108 (3S)
2SS: 2AS	24	⎬ 81 (4S)		1SS: 2AS: 1AA	48	⎬	
1SS: 3AS	32	⎬		3AS: 1AA	32	⎭	
4AS	16	⎭					
				2SS: 2AA	6	⎫	
1SS: 3AA	4	⎫		1AS: 1SS: 2AA	24	⎬	54 (2S)
1AS: 3AA	8	⎬ 12 (1S)		2AS: 2AA	24	⎭	
4AA	1		1 (0S)				

If we are surveying for the presence of sickle cell anemia, that is, for children with one or two S genes, we find through pooling of data from all the AS × AS families with four children (S = child having at least one sickle cell gene; A = child having all normal genes):

Type of sibling relationship	Number of families	S, sib	A, sib
4S	81	324	0
3S:1A	108	324	108
2S:2A	54	108	108
1S:3A	12	12	36
4A	1	0	4
	Total	768	256

This gives us the expected 3:1 ratio.

Frequently the geneticist dealing with rare diseases may not be able to distinguish between the homozygotes and the heterozygotes. This is true for sickle cell anemia, if he uses sickling as the criterion. Imagine that he decides to study AS × AA couples with four children. He would locate sickling children (as parents are normal), ignoring families with only normal children. He would necessarily also discard families with four sickling children on the assumption that they may have SS × AA parents. He would obtain a ratio of 444S:252A.

If the method of detection is the presence of hemoglobin S, the disease behaves as transmitted by a dominant trait. Thus for AA × AS couples, the geneticist expects a ratio of 1 AA child : 1 AS child. If the investigation is carried out by selecting families that have two children, one of whom is AS, then the other would be either AA or AS. Among the two-child families, there will be one family with two AS children for every two families with just one AS sib (since the children could be in the order AS-AA or AA-AS). Pooling all the children from these families, he would then find a ratio of 1 AA : 2 AS. If instead he uses another approach, such as looking for S children, and then selects those that have one sib, families with two AS children will have a double probability of being discovered. The data would then contain two AS-AS sib groups for one AS-AA sib group, and the resulting ratio would be 1 AA : 3 AS.

Let us imagine that the geneticist surveys for sickle cell anemia (or another recessive disease) and considers only the SS children:

Families with SS Children	Anemic	Normal
1 family with 4SS	4	0
12 families with 3SS	36	12
54 families with 2SS	108	108
108 families with 1SS	108	324
81 families with 0SS		324

so that the pooled data gives 256 anemic children and 728 normal children, i.e., a ratio of 1S:3A.

Surveys of recessive disease are done by locating the afflicted children, the reason being that parents are frequently normal. In this type of survey the 324 normal children would not be counted. To compensate for this, data are frequently corrected to the expected ratio by the use of suitable mathematical formulas. A significance test is performed to determine whether the probability of the ratio found matches the expected theoretical one. If there is a high probability (99 percent or more), the results are considered highly significant.

LABORATORY INVESTIGATION: HUMAN GENETICS

Prepare a pool of data from pedigrees, using collective data from your class, on taste blindness or tongue rolling.

Couple		Total	+ Children			− Children		
Type	Number	Children	No. Found	%	No. Expected	No. Found	%	No. Expected
+ +								
+ −								
− −								
Total								

Find the percentage of + and − children (that is, children with and without the trait being tested for) in the total sample. If you assume this characteristic not to be hereditary, you can expect the same percentage independently of the traits held by the parents. Calculate the expected number of + and − children, and complete the table. Use the chi-square method (Appendix VI) to test the hypothesis of noninheritance of this trait.

GENETIC COUNSELING

If a normal couple has a child with thalassemia, we know that both parents must be heterozygous for the gene, since it is inherited as a recessive. We can state that there is 1 chance in 4 that their children will have this trait. As we have seen, the fact that they have already had one child with thalassemia does not decrease the chance that subsequent children will be affected: the probability remains at 25 percent (Fig. 4-5).

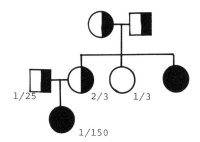

Fig. 4-5. Expectancy of thalassemia in the offspring of a couple with one affected child.

It is important to tell such couples that two-thirds of their normal children may be carriers of this abnormal trait. The chance of affected grandchildren, of course, depends on the chance of the children's meeting other carriers. In some regions of Italy the probability that the gene for thalassemia will occur is quite high, 1/25. (Generally, abnormal genes are not that common.) In this case the chance for a grandchild with thalassemia is $2/3 \times 1/25 \times 1/4 = 1/150$ (Fig. 4-5).

Let us imagine that a normal woman, with a brother who has thalassemia, decides to marry a cousin. She has a two-thirds probability of being a carrier. Her mother is a carrier and therefore must have received the gene from one of the grandparents. The grandparent has 1 chance in 2 of having given the same gene to the aunt. The aunt has 1 chance in 2 of having transmitted the disease to the cousin. Therefore the chance of affected children is $2/3 \times 1/2 \times 1/2 \times 1/4 = 1/24$ (Fig. 4-6).

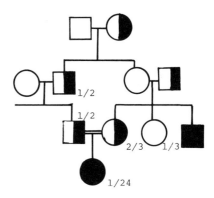

Fig. 4-6. Expectancy of thalassemia in the offspring of two cousins, one of whose parents has thalassemia.

If, instead, she decides to marry a person with an affected brother, the chance increases still further to $2/3 \times 2/3 \times 1/4 = 1/9$ (Fig. 4-7).

Counseling then, can make a very great difference, assuming the carrier can be detected. This is possible in sickle cell anemia and in several other hereditary traits. There is still very little one can do, however, apart from counseling, in cases of sickle cell anemia. It was found recently that potassium cyanate, KOCN, can reverse sickling by combining with hemoglobin and changing its properties. Since KOCN is toxic, however, it is hoped that other compounds will be developed.

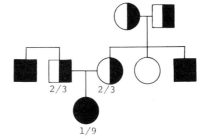

Fig. 4-7. Expectancy of thalassemia in the offspring of a couple having thalassemic sibs on both sides.

GENETIC CONTROL OF HEMOGLOBIN SYNTHESIS

Man has the potential to produce five different hemoglobin chains. These combine spontaneously to form four-chain molecules. In very early embryos, only epsilon chains are produced. These assemble to form Gower II hemoglobin. Soon alpha chain synthesis begins, and Gower I hemoglobin appears. In fetal life, epsilon production is replaced by gamma production, forming fetal hemoglobin. This persists for a few months after birth. A few months before birth, beta chains begin to be synthesized, forming hemoglobin A. The delta chain is also produced in small amounts, resulting in hemoglobin A_2. Those two hemoglobins will remain in the body for the rest of the life of the living being.

Hemoglobin	Chains
Gower II	4 epsilon
Gower I	2 alpha and 2 epsilon
Fetal	2 alpha and 2 gamma
A_2	2 alpha and 2 delta
A	2 alpha and 2 beta

Abnormalities of Hemoglobin Chains

Today about 100 hemoglobins are known that, like sickle cell hemoglobin, have one abnormal chain. The reason for this in most cases is that one amino acid has been replaced. These genes producing the normal and abnormal chains are codominant: the heterozygote has both normal and abnormal hemoglobin, and the homozygote just abnormal hemoglobin.

When there is a severe deficiency of gas transportation due to abnormal hemoglobin, the organism compensates through the production of larger amounts of hemoglobin A_2 or the production, in the adult, of fetal hemoglobin. This is what occurs in beta-thalassemia. Here there is a genetic impairment of the production of beta chains.

Determination of Abnormal Hemoglobin

The establishment of hereditary control of hemoglobin synthesis has come about through the study of pedigrees. The blood of all families being studied is collected and is examined by electrophoresis. When an unknown abnormal hemoglobin is found, it is split into chains. The isolated alpha chain is combined in vitro with a normal beta chain, and the beta chain with a normal alpha chain. Comparison of the hybrid hemoglobins with normal hemoglobin shows whether the defect is in the alpha or in the beta chain. Hydrolysis and chromatography permit identification of the specific structural defects.

Here are some examples of abnormal hemoglobins:

Hemoglobin	Defective Chain	Defective Position	Normal Amino Acid Replacement
S	beta	A_3	Glu Val
C	beta	A_3	Glu Lys
E	beta	B_8	Glu Lys
Memphis	alpha	B_8	Glu Gln
B_2	delta	A_{13}	Gly Ala

Genetic information is obtained from rare individuals or families who have one or more abnormal hemoglobins. (See Figures 4-8 through 4-13.)

From the pedigrees in Figures 4-8 through 4-13, what can be said about the inheritance of hemoglobins? How many genes could be postulated to explain it?

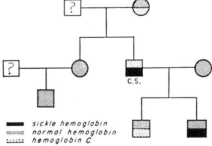

Fig. 4-8. Family with hemo-globins S and C. (Courtesy of H. M. Ranney, D. L. Larson, and G. H. McCormak, Jr. *J. Clin. Invest.* 32:1227, 1953.)

■■■ sickle hemoglobin
▨▨▨ normal hemoglobin
▦▦▦ hemoglobin C

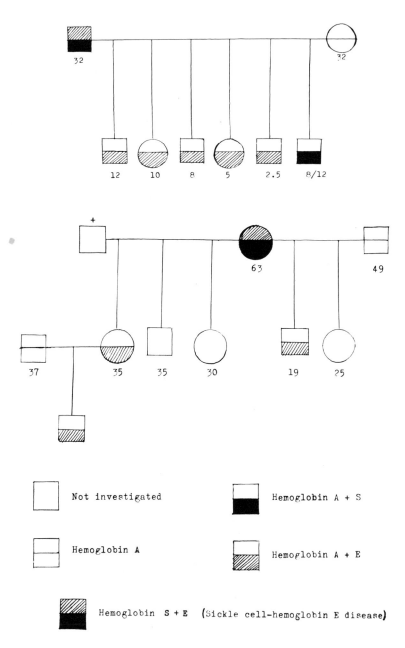

Fig. 4-9. Family pedigrees with hemoglobins S and E. (Courtesy of M. Aksoy, *Blood* 15:610, 1960.)

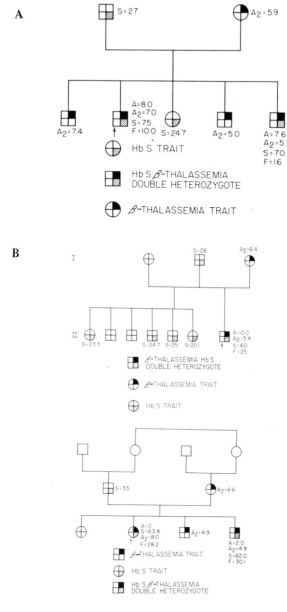

A

S=27   A₂=5.9

A=8.0
A₂=7.0
S=75
F=10.0   S=24.7

A₂=7.4   ↑   Hb S TRAIT   A₂=5.0   A=7.6
                                         A₂=5.7
                                         S=70
                                         F=16

Hb S β-THALASSEMIA
DOUBLE HETEROZYGOTE

β-THALASSEMIA TRAIT

B

I   S=26   A₂=6.4

II   A=10.0
   S=23.3   S=24.7 S=25 S=201   A₂=5.4
                                    S=60
                                    F=25

β-THALASSEMIA HbS
DOUBLE HETEROZYGOTE

β-THALASSEMIA TRAIT

Hb S TRAIT

S=33   A₂=6.6

          A=0   A=2.0
          S=63.8   A₂=4.9
          A₂=8.0   A₂=4.9   S=62.0
          F=28.2   F=30.1

β-THALASSEMIA TRAIT

Hb S TRAIT

Hb S β-THALASSEMIA
DOUBLE HETEROZYGOTE

Fig. 4-10. Family pedigree with hemoglobin S and beta-thalassemia. (Courtesy of J. R. McNiel, *Am. J. Hum. Genet.* 18:100, 1967. Copyright © 1967 by The University of Chicago.)

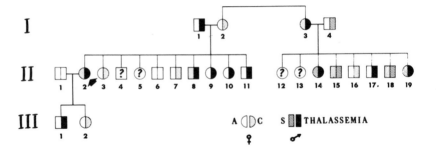

Fig. 4-11. Family pedigree with hemoglobin C and beta-thalassemia. (Courtesy of P. R. McCurdy, and H. A. Pearson, *Am. J. Hum. Genet.* 13:390, 1961. Copyright © 1961 by The University of Chicago.)

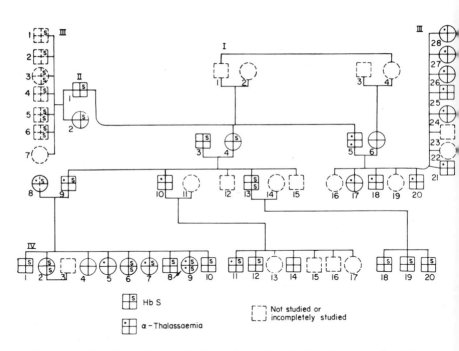

Fig. 4-12. Family pedigree with hemoglobin S and alpha-thalassemia. (Courtesy of D. J. Weatherall, J. B. Clegg, J. Blankson, and J. R. McNiel, *Br. J. Haematol.* 17:517, 1969.)

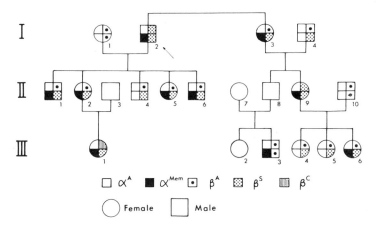

Fig. 4-13. Family pedigree with hemoglobins S, C, and Memphis. (Courtesy of L. M. Kraus, T. Miayaji, I. Iuchi, and A. P. Draus, *Biochemistry* 5:3701, 1966.)

Genetic Control in Abnormal Hemoglobin

It seems logical to postulate one gene controlling the biosynthesis of each hemoglobin chain. This would explain why in beta-thalassemia, although the synthesis of the beta chain is impaired, A_2 and F hemoglobins may be produced at higher rates. In alpha-thalassemia the alpha chain biosynthesis is the one impaired. Therefore, the four beta chains associate to form H hemoglobin, and in the case of the fetus the four gamma chains associate to form Barth hemoglobin.

The pedigrees show that, as one would expect, E, C, S, and normal beta genes are alleles. Memphis is an allele to the normal alpha chain gene. As seen in Figure 4-13, it is possible for one person to possess four hemoglobins if he is heterozygous for the genes for both the alpha and the beta chains. This could occur as follows:

	alpha	alpha^{Mem}
beta	A	Mem
beta S	S	S-Mem

We do not have fully detailed information on the genetic control of hemoglobin biosynthesis. In some rare families, fetal hemoglobin occurs in the normal adult. There seems to be a genetic lack of control that fails to stop production of gamma chains in adult life. This leads us to postulate the existence of an additional set of genes, a set which controls the genes that determine the several chains. These control genes would be responsible for the shutting on and off of the chain-producing genes. Thalassemia could be the result of abnormal control genes for either alpha or beta chains.

Genes and Chromosomes

Study the pedigree of the family that has both S and B_2 (abnormal delta chain, symbolized as A^1_2) hemoglobins (Fig. 4-14). One woman (II-5) has four different hemoglobins, A,S, A_2, and B_2, and by three marriages has eight children. The hemoglobins of two husbands are not known but can be assumed to be normal A,A_2. What possible descendants can be expected theoretically? Are all combinations fulfilled?

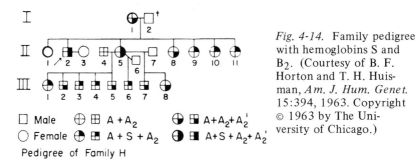

Fig. 4-14. Family pedigree with hemoglobins S and B_2. (Courtesy of B. F. Horton and T. H. Huisman, *Am. J. Hum. Genet.* 15:394, 1963. Copyright © 1963 by The University of Chicago.)

The human adult has about 20,000 genes, of which fewer than 2,000 have been identified. We know that these genes are located on chromosomes and come in pairs. We may suppose that each gene is located at a very specific point on a certain chromosome. Since there are two chromosomes for each pair, the second may contain the same gene as the first (homozygote) or it may contain an allele (heterozygote). One of each pair is transmitted, through either sperm cells or eggs, to the descendants.

Now imagine a species with just two pairs of chromosomes. One doubly heterozygous individual could have chromosome pairs as shown in Figure 4-15. The sperm (or eggs) could have chromosomes carrying either AB, Ab, aB, or ab. It is evident that, on crossing this individual with another of similar genetic constitution, we would get a recombination of the two genes in the proportions expected by Mendel's laws.

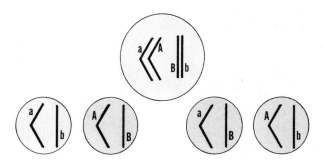

Fig. 4-15. Segregation of genes by assortment of chromosomes during gamete formation. Top: genotype. Bottom: gametes.

In the case of genes located on the same chromosome (linked) (Fig. 4-16), one would not expect all four combinations, but just aC or Ac. Does this explain the results in the previous pedigree (Fig. 4-14)?

Fig. 4-16. Gene linkage.

Horton and Huisman reviewed the cases published up to 1963 and found the following:*

Author	AA_2	SA_2	AB_2	SB_2
Cepellini (1959)	0	4	2	0
Horton et al. (1961)	0	1	4	0
Raney et al. (1963)	0	2	3	0
	0	2	1	0
	0	3	1	0
Horton and Huisman (1963)	0	4	4	0
Total	0	16	13	0

Applying the chi-square method in a small number of cases, they found a probability of less than 0.01 that the lack of recombination of the abnormal chains is accidental.

*Table reprinted from Horton, B. F., and Huisman, T. H. *Am. J. Hum. Genet.* 15:394 (1963). Copyright © 1963 by The University of Chicago, 1963.

In the same journal, around the same time three more pedigrees were published. These are shown in Figure 4-17. Include the data from them in the table above, and recalculate the probability.

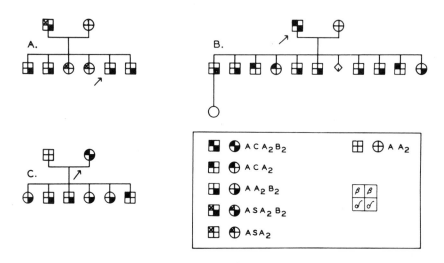

Fig. 4-17. Family pedigrees with hemoglobins S and B_2. (Courtesy of S. H. Boyer, D. L. Rucknagel, D. J. Weatherall, and E. J. Watson-Williams, *Am. J. Hum. Genet.* 15:438, 1963. Copyright © 1963 by The University of Chicago.)

Examine the pedigree in Figure 4-18, especially the child of couple II 2-3. Does it conform to the phenomenon of linkage?

It is clear that the genes for the B_2 trait come from the grandfather's family and for the beta-thalassemia, from the grandmother's family. They must be on different chromosomes. III-2, however, has both abnormal traits. This suggests that the two abnormal genes became located on the same chromosome.

Figure 4-19 is an example of a pair of chromosomes exchanging pieces — a phenomenon known as *crossing-over.* For B_2 and beta-thalassemia genes, the available data show this happening in 7 percent of the cases. Other genes studied have a higher frequency of recombination. In order for crossing-over to occur in chromosomes, the chromosome chain must break at some point. If two particular genes on a chromosome are very far apart, the chance for the break's occurring between them is greater than if they are very close together. Therefore, beta-thalassemia and B_2 genes (or their normal counterparts) must be very close together.

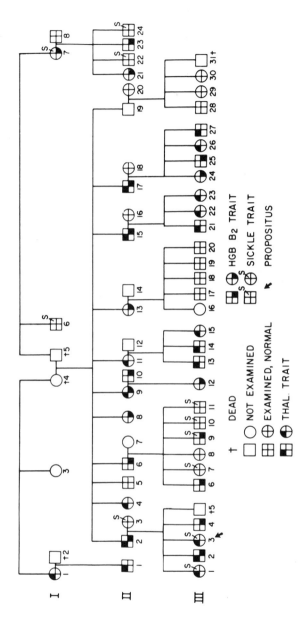

Fig. 4-18. Family pedigree with hemoglobins S and B₂. (Courtesy of H. A. Pearson and M. M. Moore, *Am. J. Hum. Genet.* 17:125, 1965. Copyright © 1965 by The University of Chicago.)

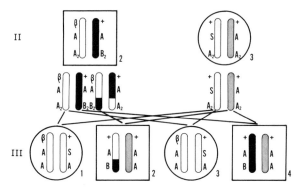

Fig. 4-19. Recombination of hemoglobins A, S, A_2, and B_2 by crossing-over.

Delta and beta genes must be even closer, since recombinants are never found. This agrees with the discovery of a very strange hemoglobin called *hemoglobin lepore*. Hemoglobin lepore is found in patients with normal beta and delta chains, and therefore normal A and A_2 hemoglobins, but with a new chain consisting of part beta and part delta chains. Apparently an abnormal break took place in the middle of a beta gene on one chromosome and in a delta gene on the other. Then through a process of exchange a hybrid beta-delta gene is produced (Fig. 4-20).

Studies on the evolution of hemoglobin suggest that the primitive vertebrates, such as the lamprey, had only a single chain hemoglobin, controlled by a single gene. This gene must have duplicated to create the alpha and beta chains and again to produce the gamma and delta genes (Fig. 4-21). These duplications probably occurred through asymmetrical crossing-over which left one chromosome with two genes. Once duplicated, one gene would continue to produce the same hemoglobin chain. The other could undergo evolutionary changes to make a new chain.

Height and skin color are obvious hereditary traits. But one finds a continuous variation between two extremes. This cannot be explained by a single pair of genes, which without dominance give three discrete phenotypes — AA, Aa, and aa. It can be explained, however, by postulating a number of alleles, with equal function. With two pairs of alleles, for example, there are five phenotypes:

AABB	AaBB	AaBb	Aabb	aabb
	AABb	AAbb	aaBb	
		aaBB		

Data for skin color fit a five-pair allele system.

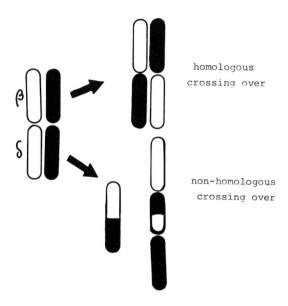

homologous
crossing over

non-homologous
crossing over

Fig. 4-20. Homologous and nonhomologous crossing-over.

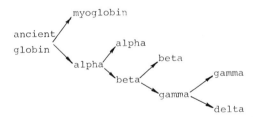

Fig. 4-21. Evolution of hemoglobin chains by gene duplication.

SEX-LINKED TRAITS

Some families present, as a hereditary trait, a susceptibility to hemolytic
anemia when they breathe the pollen of broad beans *(Vicia faba)* or take drugs
such as sulfanilamide or primaquine (for the cure or prevention of malaria).
Examining the pedigrees of these families shows that the disease is more common among females, who may present either a mild or a severe form. Males,
on the other hand, present only the severe form. The transmission of this trait
shows:

severely affected female × normal male: mildly affected females

affected males

mildly affected female × normal male: half of the females mildly affected

half of the males affected

affected male × normal female: no affected males

mildly affected females

How can this be explained?

The existence of mild and severe forms in the female suggests that the trait is transmitted by a codominant gene. The severe cases are homozygous and the mild cases heterozygous.

Sex is known to be determined by a special pair of chromosomes, the *sex chromosomes.* In the female these consist of a pair of X-chromosomes. In the male there is one X-chromosome and a smaller chromosome called a *Y-chromosome* (Fig. 4-22). The inheritance of anemia can be explained easily if one assumes that the gene is located on the X-chromosome. Let us represent the abnormal allele for primaquine anemia by a G, and the normal allele by an N. Females may be either $X^N X^N$, $X^G X^N$, or $X^G X^G$, and males $X^N Y$ or $X^G Y$.

Sex-linked traits have been known for many centuries. The Jews, who practiced circumcision, knew about *hemophilia* or the *bleeder disease,* and had a set of rules which applied to children from families that had this trait. The gene for hemophilia is rare, and it is recessive to the normal allele. It is exceptionally rare to find hemophilic females, who must be homozygous for the abnormal gene.

Try to establish rules for the presence of hemophilic grandchildren when the grandfather has the trait.

It is evident that a hemophiliac can transmit the trait only to his daughters. They are carriers but are otherwise normal. The granddaughters also are carriers, whereas half the grandsons are bleeders.

Several abnormal genes and their normal alleles have been traced to the X-chromosome, examples being color blindness, hemophilia, vitamin D—resistant rickets, muscular dystrophy, and brown-enameled teeth. These are not genes related to sexual functions; therefore it seems strange that the female would have two genes for each characteristic, and the male just one.

In 1961 Mary Lyon proposed that one of the female's X-chromosomes becomes inactivated in a random way. If this hypothesis is correct, one could

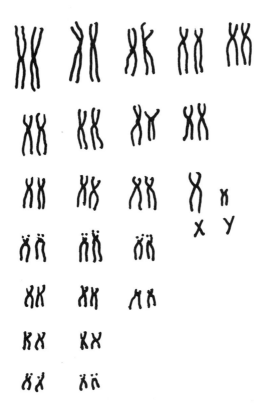

Fig. 4-22. A set of male human chromosomes.

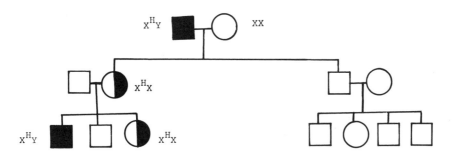

Fig. 4-23. Sex-linked inheritance. H = hemophilic gene.

expect in the case of primaquine anemia in the heterozygous female a mixture of normal and sensitive red cells. This has been proved to be correct, as is shown in the paper at the end of this chapter.

GROUP DISCUSSION: GENETIC COUNSELING

Is there genetic counseling available in the local community? Who uses it?

How much do people in the community know about hereditary disease? Has the school system any role in educating them about it?

What are the superstitions and traditions of the community in relation to hereditary diseases and malformations?

Would you tell a couple, "You have a chance in four of having an abnormal child" or, "your chance of having a normal child is three out of four"?

In advising parents, would you take into consideration the economic burden of an abnormal child? What are the social facilities for helping abnormal children in the community?

Is your role as a doctor to inform, advise, or interfere?

Would you advise a couple to use artificial insemination from a sperm bank? When?

Would you advise, and when would you advise, an abortion?

What is the legal status of some of these measures?

The role of the counselor is simplest in the case of single genes or chromosomal defects. Many diseases, however, have a hereditary and a nonhereditary component, like diabetes, and for many there are complex genetic mechanisms. What is the role of the counselor in these cases?

SELF-EVALUATION

1. A man marries a woman who is not related to him, and their first son has albinism, a defect in skin pigmentation transmitted by a recessive gene.
   a. The chance that the next child will be an albino is
   b. The chance of their having four albino children is
   c. The chance that this son's first son will carry the gene is
   (choose one answer for each of the above)
   p. 1:3.
   q. 3:1.
   r. 50 percent.
   s. 25 percent.
   t. 6.25 percent.
   u. very small.

2. If a man who is affected by primaquine sensitivity marries a woman who is normal,
   a. only daughters will carry the gene.
   b. only sons will carry the gene.
   c. both sons and daughters will carry the gene.
   d. there is no probability, as this is not a genetic disease.

3. Primaquine sensitivity is transmitted by an X-linked gene. We can suppose that the disease
   a. is practically limited to men.
   b. has doubled incidence in women.
   c. has about the same incidence in both sexes.

   To explain each of these three possibilities we must suppose that the gene is
   p. dominant.
   q. recessive.
   r. codominant.
   s. partly inactivated, as one X-chromosome is inactivated in the female.

4. A man with hemoglobins S and E is accused of being the father of a child of a woman with normal hemoglobin. The child has normal hemoglobin only.
   a. The man is probably the father.
   b. The man cannot be the father.
   c. It is impossible to know from these data.

5. The frequency of a gene is 0.01. How much higher is the chance for a defective offspring if a carrier of this gene marries a cousin?

THE SEPARATION OF GLUCOSE-6-PHOSPHATE-DEHYDRO-GENASE-DEFICIENT ERYTHROCYTES FROM THE BLOOD OF HETEROZYGOTES FOR GLUCOSE-6-PHOSPHATE-DEHYDROGENASE DEFICIENCY*

Ernest Beutler‡, Maryellen C. Baluda§

In 1960 Ohno et al. demonstrated that the two X-chromosomes of females of various mammalian species were different (Ohno and Hauschka 1960, Ohno and Makino 1961). One was hyperpyknotic and formed the chromatin body, while the other resembled the autosomes. This observation led Lyon (1961), who was working with sex-linked coat-colour genes, to suggest that the hyperpyknotic X-chromosome was genetically inactive, that inactivation took place in early embryonic life, and that the same X-chromosome remained inactivated in the progeny of each cell of the embryo once inactivation had taken place.

We had independently formulated the same hypothesis, on the basis of Ohno's observations, to explain certain troublesome features regarding the genetics of a sex-linked mutation of man—glucose-6-phosphate-dehydrogenase (G.-6-P.D.) deficiency (Beutler 1962). We reasoned that if one of the X-chromosomes of the female heterozygote was inactivated, then females with intermediate enzyme activity in the peripheral blood should have two red-cell populations. These would consist of one population of enzyme-deficient red cells, and one population of normal red cells. The disappearance of glutathione from these cells when challenged with acetylphenylhydrazine, and the reduction of methaemoglobin in them, was found to occur in two components. The curves obtained were virtually identical with those obtained with artificial mixtures of normal and enzyme-deficient red cells (Beutler et al. 1962). Attempts to demonstrate by histochemical means that two cell populations were present were technically unsatisfactory (Beutler 1962, Beutler and Fairbanks 1962, Beutler et al. 1962).

We have now succeeded in separating enzyme-deficient red cells from the blood of Negro women who are heterozygous for G.-6-P.D. deficiency. This was accomplished by studying the red cells of a subject who was heterozygous for this abnormality and for sickle-cell haemoglobin. Since the sickle-cell trait does not measurably shorten the lifespan of erythrocytes, these cells may be considered in every way comparable to cells from other heterozygotes for G.-6-P.D. deficiency, but the presence of sickle haemoglobin made it possible to separate the cells with a high proportion of methaemoglobin (enzyme-deficient cells) from those with a low proportion of methaemoglobin (normal cells). This could be accomplished because methaemoglobin-containing sickle cells will not undergo sickling when the oxygen tension is decreased (Itano 1950, Beutler 1961).

*This paper was presented, in part, at the IXth European Congress of Haematology, in August, 1963. Beutler, Dern, and Baluda (1963).
‡M.D. Chicago, Chairman, Department of Medicine, City of Hope Medical Center; Associate Clinical Professor of Medicine, University of Southern California
§M.S. Pittsburg, Research Technician, Department of Medicine, City of Hope Medical Center

METHODS
Subjects

Two Negro women with the sickle-cell trait and with intermediate red-cell G.-6-P.D. levels, therefore presumably heterozygous for G.-6-P.D. deficiency (subjects no. 1 and 2), one subject with the sickle trait but with a normal red-cell G.-6-P.D. level (subject no. 3), and two normal subjects (subjects no. 4 and 5) were studied. 8 ml. of blood was drawn into 2 ml. acid-citrate-dextrose (N.I.H. formula B) and stored at 4°C before use. All studies were carried out within 24 hours of taking the blood samples.

Oxidation of Haemoglobin by Nitrite and its Reduction

The blood sample was centrifuged, the plasma was removed, and the cells were treated with 1% sodium-nitrite solution to convert their haemoglobin to methaemoglobin. The buffy coat was removed and the red cells were washed five times in 7–10 volumes of 0.9% NaCl solution. They were then incubated in a system containing glucose and Nile-blue sulphate. This system has been described in detail elsewhere (Beutler and Baluda 1963, Beutler et al. 1963). It permits normal erythrocytes to reduce methaemoglobin rapidly, but allows G.-6-P.D.-deficient cells to do so only very slowly. There is no interaction between normal and enzyme-deficient red cells; each cell reduces methaemoglobin at a rate which is closely related to its G.-6-P.D. activity (Beutler and Baluda 1963).

Millipore-filtration Studies

These were carried out by a modification of the method of Jandl et al. (1961). Plasma from a compatible donor was used as a suspending medium for the sickling of red cells and their subsequent filtration. It was prepared from blood drawn into ethylenediamine tetra-acetic acid and freed of suspended material by high-speed centrifugation and millipore filtration (Jandl et al. 1961). Plasma stored in the frozen state before use was found preferable to fresh plasma because the nonspecific methaemoglobin-reducing action (Beutler and Baluda 1963) of such plasma was less. After use, the suspending plasma was recovered, reprocessed, and reused.

A 45 mm. millipore-filter disc, with a mean pore size of 5 μ, was employed in these studies. The filtration assembly was prepared by thoroughly moistening the sintered glass portion with 0.9% NaCl solutions, and placing the filter disc into position while moistened with saline solution. The top of the inflow assembly was sealed with a rubber disc, and the space above the filter was flushed out thoroughly with the water-saturated 10% CO_2/90% nitrogen gas mixture employed. Hypodermic needles were pushed through the rubber disc for this purpose, as suggested to us by Dr. J. H. Jandl. The filter disc was moistened with plasma just before filtration of the cell mixture. Filtration was carried out under a pressure of 82 mm. Hg.

Preliminary studies with this system indicated that virtually no deoxygenated cells from a sickle-trait (S.-A.) subject passed through the millipore filter. If a mixture of equal numbers of S.-A. cells and normal cells was passed through the filter, each at a concentration of 0.15%, slightly over half of the normal cells passed the filter up to a suspension volume of 15 ml. At higher volumes, the passage of a large proportion of normal cells was impeded in the presence of sickle cells, presumably because the cells clogged the filter pores.

Microdeterminations of G.-6-P.D. and Methaemoglobin

G.-6-P.D. activity was measured by a micro-adaptation of the method of Marks (1958).† The concentration of glucose-6-phosphate was reduced to 0.05 M. This does not affect the enzyme activity (Beutler 1960). The volume of all other reactants was reduced to 1/10 of the usual quantity except that either 5 or 10 μ litres of haemolysate was used. Assays were carried out in the Zeiss PMQ II spectrophotometer, using a microcuvette with a critical volume of approximately 0.24 ml. and a path length of 1.000 cm. The results were expressed as optical density (O.D.) units per gramme haemoglobin, as referred to the usual 2.5 ml. assay system. In effect, this was achieved by dividing enzyme activity by 10, to compensate for the reduced distribution volume of the haemolysate.

In carrying out methaemoglobin determinations the same micro-cuvettes were employed. A slit-width of 0.02–0.05 mm. on the monochrometer of PMQ II spectrophotometer was found to be satisfactory. Methaemoglobin and haemoglobin determinations were carried out by a micromodification of the method of Evelyn and Malloy (1938). 0.3 ml. of $M/60$ phosphate buffer, pH 6.6, containing 0.02% saponin was placed into each microcuvette. 20 μ litres of haemolysate was added, and an O.D. reading was made against a water blank at 630 mμ (reading A). 5 μ litres of neutralised 5% sodium-cyanide solution was added to the cuvette; it was mixed, and a second reading was taken at 630 mμ (reading B). 5 μ litres of 5% potassium-ferricyanide solution was then added to the same cuvette, and the optical density at 540 mμ was determined (reading C). The methaemoglobin and haemoglobin concentrations were computed as follows, on the basis of factors derived from methaemoglobin solutions of known concentrations:

$$\text{Methaemoglobin (\% of total pigment)} = \left(\frac{0.98\ A - B}{C}\right)323.$$

Total haemoglobin (mg. per ml.) = 23.3C.

The factor 0.98 was applied to the A reading to compensate for the fall in O.D. produced by a dilution of the 0.320 ml. haemoglobin solution by the 5 μ litres of the cyanide solution.

EXPERIMENTS

The reduction of methaemoglobin in the red cells from the five subjects in the Nile-blue-containing incubation system is presented in the figure. The cells from both subjects with intermediate G.-6-P.D. activity reduced methaemoglobin in two components, as we have previously shown to be typical for subjects heterozygous for G.-6-P.D. deficiency (Beutler et al. 1962, 1963). At the end of 3 hours, an aliquot was removed from the incubation system containing cells from heterozygotes for G.-6-P.D. deficiency; in the other cases the aliquot was taken when the methaemoglobin level had fallen to between 35% and 45%. The aliquot was immediately chilled in ice and washed twice in cold 0.9% sodium-chloride solution. Slightly more than 13 ml. of a 0.15% red-cell

† Normal values (mean ± 1 S.D.) = 15.9 ± 2.4. Negro G.-6-P.D. deficient hemizygote (mean ± 1 S.D.) = 2.7 ± 1.5.

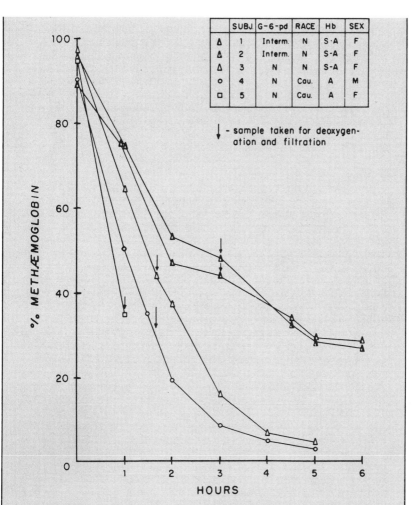

	SUBJ.	G-6-pd	RACE	Hb	SEX
Δ	1	Interm.	N	S·A	F
Δ	2	Interm.	N	S·A	F
Δ	3	N	N	S·A	F
o	4	N	Cau.	A	M
□	5	N	Cau.	A	F

↓ – sample taken for deoxygen-
ation and filtration

The reduction of methaemoglobin in the nitrite-treated red cells of the five subjects studied. The incubation system described in detail previously (Beutler and Báluda, 1963) contained glucose, buffer, and Nile-blue sulphate in addition to the erythrocytes. The two-component nature of the methaemoglobin-reduction curves obtained from the heterozygous subjects is clearly evident.

suspension in plasma was exposed to a mixture of water-saturated 10% carbon dioxide/90% nitrogen for 20 minutes, by rotating at room temperature in a sealed separatory funnel which was repeatedly flushed with the gas mixture. 10 ml. of the cell suspension was then transferred anaerobically to the millipore-filter assembly; the upper chamber had been equilibrated with 10% CO_2/90% N. The suspension was then filtered at 82 mm. Hg, the filter was changed, and a second 13 ml. aliquot was treated in the same manner.

The red-cell suspension passing the millipore filter was centrifuged, and the small button of red cells obtained was washed once in 0.9% NaCl solution. Simultaneously, the red cells from an accurately measured 3–4 ml. aliquot of the gassed but unfiltered 0.15% red-cell suspension were separated by centrifugation and washed. Each sample of cells was haemolysed by freezing and thawing twice. Using micropipettes, the haemolysate was transferred to another iced test-tube, and the total volume was accurately adjusted to between 110 and 150 μ litres. The haemoglobin and methaemoglobin content and G.-6-P.D. activity of all samples was then determined.

RESULTS

The results of these studies are shown in the table. When cell suspensions were prepared from the double heterozygotes (no. 1 and 2) the non-sickled forms passing the filter had a very high methaemoglobin content and a low enzyme activity. The filtered cells contained 2.34 and 2.56 units of activity per gramme haemoglobin. This is less enzyme activity than is found in the red cells of the average affected male hemizygote – i.e., 2.7 units per g. haemoglobin (Marks and Gross 1959). The low enzyme activity found in the cells passing the filter is not a result of their manipulation, since normal erythrocytes (no. 5 and 6) lost no enzyme activity when carried through the same process. Further, this difference could not merely be a manifestation of red-cell age. Because younger red cells have a greater capacity to reduce methaemoglobin than have older cells (Jung 1949, Lohr et al. 1958, Jalavisto and Solantera 1959), filtration exerted some selective influence on the red cells of the subject with a sickle trait but with normal G.-6-P.D. (no. 3). This selective influence, however, was quite small. The difference between the methaemoglobin content of the mixed cells and of the filtered cells, as well as the difference in enzyme activity between the mixed cells and the filtered cells was less than 20%. Undoubtedly, this is a function of red-cell age.

In each case the methaemoglobin concentration in the mixed plasma-suspended cells was somewhat lower than the concentration of methaemoglobin at the time an aliquot was removed from the Nile-blue-containing incubation mixture (see table). This can undoubtedly be accounted for by the non-specific methaemoglobin-reducing activity of plasma on red-cell suspensions (Beutler and Baluda 1963). In previous studies we found that after 3 hours' incubation of red cells of hemizygous G.-6-P.D. deficient males in the system used, methaemoglobin levels were 65 to 80% (Beutler et al. 1963). The slightly lower levels encountered in the filtered cells from female heterozygotes (63% and 60%) are readily accounted for by the non-specific methaemoglobin-reducing effect of plasma. It is quite clear, therefore, that the cells obtained through filtration of the treated blood of double heterozygotes resembled in every way the cells of hemizygous males, and it is quite important that the cells were obtained in relatively high yield. This excludes the possibility that these were a relatively few cells representing one tail of a normal distribution curve.

DISCUSSION

The evidence for inactivation of an X-chromosome in the normal human female is quite incomplete. Yet, the problems of dosage effect

THE RESULTS

Subject No.	1		2		3		4		5	
Race/sex	N/F		N/F		N/F		C/M		C/F	
Hb type/G.-6-P.D.	S.-A./intermediate		S.-A./intermediate		S.-A./normal		A./normal		A./normal	
	MHb (%)	G.-6-P.D. (U per g.Hb)	MHb (%)	G.-6-P.D. (U per g.Hb)	MHb (%)	G.-6-P.D. (U per g.Hb)	MHb (%)	G.-6-P.D. (U per g.Hb)	MHb (%)	G.-6-P.D. (U per g.Hb)
Original red blood-cells (R.B.C.s)	1.35	6.35	0.74	7.31	3.90	15.99	2.07	12.65	0	10.69
R.B.C.s at time of removal from Nile-blue incubation system (see figure)	44.7	...	48.7	...	44.2	...	32.8	...	35.6	...
Plasma suspended R.B.C.s (after nitrite treatment and partial methaemoglobin reduction)	27.6	6.61	38.3	7.92	37.63	15.14	19.17	12.91	26.96	11.02
R.B.C.s passing filter	60.4	2.34	63.3	2.56	45.89	13.26	18.35	12.93	20.01	10.32
Yield (% passing filter)	19%		27%		26%		67%		45%	

N = Negro, C = Caucasian, MHb = methaemoglobin.

involving the X-chromosome and the greatly varied expression of certain
X-linked traits in the female are very nicely explained by this hypothesis.

Some evidence in favour of inactivation of at least some of the loci of
the human X-chromosome has been presented. The locus for G.-6-P.D.
deficiency is one of those most suitable for investigation. We originally
demonstrated that the rate of methaemoglobin reduction and the rate of
destruction of reduced glutathione (G.S.H.) in erythrocytes from heterozygotes for G.-6-P.D. deficiency follow a two-component curve, closely
resembling that found in artificial mixture of normal and enzyme-deficient cells (Beutler et al. 1962). We recognised that the evidence for the
existence of two red-cell populations was indirect, and that other explanations were possible. For example, a two-component curve might have
resulted from an abrupt change in enzyme activity with age, occurring at
approximately the midpoint of the life-span of the cell. This seems un-
likely, especially since one would then expect two component curves
with cells from normal subjects. It might have been supposed that the
capacity of red cells to reduce methaemoglobin would decrease considerably after 3 hours. The ability of red cells to maintain glutathione
levels, however, remains unimpaired for at least 6 hours, and the same
metabolic pathways are involved. Further, there is no decrease in the
rate of methaemoglobin reduction in enzyme-deficient cells incubated
in the same system. A "threshold-effect" may also be postulated,
wherein both the rate of methaemoglobin reduction and G.S.H. preservation does not bear a continuous linear relationship to G.-6-P.D. activity.
This would represent a most extraordinary biochemical situation.

We therefore considered the interpretation of two red-cell populations
to be by far the most likely. However, studies of the disappearance of
diisopropylfluorophosphate[32] (D.F.P.[32])-labelled red cells during drug-
induced haemolysis in heterozygotes for G.-6-P.D. deficiency were interpreted as showing that no normal red cells were present (Brewer et al.
1962). Such a conclusion seems unwarranted because:

1. The calculations made failed to take into account the fact that
only half of the enzyme-deficient cells are destroyed by drug administration (Beutler et al. 1954), and, therefore, that the cells remaining
after the episode of drug-induced haemolysis would represent a mixture of normal and enzyme-deficient cells.

2. The assumption was made that massive haemolysis of abnormal
cells would exert no influence on the survival of circulating normal cells.
In point of fact, it has been demonstrated that destruction of non-viable
cells affects the survival of circulating red cells (Jacob et al. 1962).

3. The destruction of enzyme-deficient red cells through the administration of drugs is very complex and poorly understood (Beutler 1960).
In attempting to define gene action, it is important to measure a para-
meter as close to the gene product as possible. Destruction of red cells
through the effect of drug administration is a relatively remote consequence of enzyme deficiency.

Nontheless, the D.F.P.[32] survival data have caused some doubt to be
cast upon the presence of two red-cell populations in G.-6-P.D. deficiency
(McKusick 1962, Harris 1963). It was apparent further that more direct
evidence was required to determine whether or not there were two red-
cell populations in heterozygotes for G.-6-P.D. deficiency. In the studies
reported here, it has been possible to demonstrate directly, for the first

time, that a sizeable population of grossly enzyme-deficient red cells can be isolated from the blood of subjects who are heterozygous for G.-6-P.D. deficiency. If a correction for nonspecific cell loss is made on the filter, then this accounts for approximately half of the cells. By simple subtraction it is evident that a population of red cells with normal enzyme activity must also be present.

We interpret the course of events in the double heterozygote for G.-6-P.D. deficiency and sickle-cell trait as follows. First, approximately 90% of the haemoglobin in the red cells was converted to methaemoglobin with sodium nitrite, which was then removed by washing. During incubation with Nile-blue sulphate, cells containing normal amounts of enzyme rapidly reduced their methaemoglobin so that they were virtually methaemoglobin-free at the end of 3 hours. At this time, however, enzyme-deficient red cells still contained a relatively high proportion of methaemoglobin. This was reduced slightly during suspension in plasma, but it remained at levels well over 50%. When the oxygen tension was reduced, the cells containing primarily oxyhaemoglobin underwent sickling. Cells containing a high proportion of methaemoglobin failed to sickle. When the suspension was subjected to millipore filtration, the sickled forms containing a normal amount of enzyme were held back by the filter. Undoubtedly, some unsickled forms were trapped together with the sickled forms in the filter. A high proportion of the unsickled methaemoglobin-containing cells passed the filter, however, and as would be expected if two red-cell populations were present, the cells passing the filter contained a high average proportion of methaemoglobin and contained very little G.-6-P.D. activity: they resembled entirely the red cells of the fully affected male.

Other data bearing on the inactivation of the G.-6-P.D. locus have been presented. Gartler et al. (1962) have demonstrated that tissue cultures from the skin of G.-6-P.D.-deficient subjects show decreased enzyme activity. In 1961, Gartler obtained skin-biopsy specimens from some of our patients and from other patients who were heterozygous for G.-6-P.D. deficiency; long-term culture of these cells was carried out, and the growth curves were interpreted as being compatible with the growth of a mixture of two populations of cells (Gartler 1962). Cloning was not accomplished by Gartler, but it has recently been performed by other investigators who confirmed that two types of cells were present— those with low and those with normal enzyme activity (Davidson et al. 1963).

The evidence for inactivation of loci of other sex-linked genes is less compelling. It has been pointed out that the fundus of heterozygotes for the sex-linked ocular abnormalities, choroideraemia and ocular albinism, demonstrate mosaicism (Lyon 1962). But examination of such fundi does not reveal clear-cut mosaicism showing alternation between normal and abnormal patches. Rather there is a fine mottling of the fundus which might represent mosaicism but which cannot clearly be interpreted as doing so. It has also been pointed out that the sex-linked anaemia described by Rundles and Falls (1946) fits the inactivated-X hypothesis. Female heterozygotes demonstrate small numbers of abnormal cells and large numbers of normal cells. What is disturbing is the fact that the number of abnormal cells comprise perhaps less than 5% of the total cells in the smears. This is true both in the original illustrations and in examination of smears from heterozygotes which we have had an opportunity to see, through the courtesy of Dr. Ronald Bishop. Furthermore, some female heterozygotes had normal blood but splenomegaly. These findings could be explained through much shortened survival of defective erythrocytes in the peripheral blood. However, no evidence of excessive haemolysis is apparent in the hemizygotes, all of whose cells should bear the abnormality. It is also possible that the abnormal cells in the marrow have a reduced survival value or proliferate more slowly, thus leading to gradual elimination of the mutant clone. In the case of colour blindness, another sex-linked trait, we have been unable to demonstrate mosaicism (Krill and Beutler 1964). This could have been owing to the presence of a very fine mosaic, smaller than the half-degree targets which were used in testing the retina; nonetheless, it must be conceded that the results were negative. In the case of ectodermal dysplasia, Motulsky (1962) has demonstrated alternating areas of involved and uninvolved skin. The interpretation of this data is not entirely clear, however, since hemizygous males also demonstrated some patchiness. Histological study of muscles from heterozygotes for sex-linked dystrophy has shown patches of normal and abnormal muscle (Pearson et al. 1963). Examination of the red cells of subjects heterozygous for the X-gA blood-group has failed to demonstrate mosaicism (Gorman et al. 1963). This may indicate that the entire X-chromosome is not inactivated or that the X-gA antigen is not produced by the erythroblast, or it could be due to technical factors. Nonetheless, the reported result is negative, and this has recently been confirmed (Reed et al. 1963).

In view of the somewhat equivocal results obtained when other sex-linked characteristics of man have been studied, further confirmation of inactivation of the locus for G.-6-P.D. deficiency in one of the two X-chromosomes of the female is of particular interest.

We are grateful to Dr. D. Powars, Dr. R. Day, and Dr. S. W. for making blood samples available to use for study.

This work was supported in part by a U.S. Public Health Serv. grant.

REFERENCES

Beutler, E. (1960) *in* Metabolic Basis of Inherited Disease (edited J. B. Stanbury, J. B. Wyngaarden, and D. S. Fredrickson); p.g. New York.
—   (1961) *J. Clin. Invest.* 40, 1856.
—   (1962) *in* Mechanisms of Anemia (edited by I. Weinstein and Beutler); p. 195. New York.
—   Baluda, M. C. (1963) *Blood,* 22, 323.
—   Dern, R. J., Alving, A. S. (1954) *J. Lab. Clin. Med.* 44, 439.
—   — Baluda, M. C. (1963) Proceedings of the IXth European Congress of Haematology, Lisbon (1961) (in the press).
—   Fairbanks, V. F. (1962) Proceedings of the IXth Internatl. Society of Haematology, Mexico City (in the press).
—   Yeh, M., Fairbanks, V. F. (1962) *Proc. Nat. Acad. Sci.* 48, 9.
Brewer, G. J., Tarlov, A. R., Powell, R. D. (1962) *J. Clin. Invest.* 41.
Davidson, R. G., Nitowsky, H. M., Childs, B. (1963) *Proc. Nat. Acad.* 50, 481.
Evelyn, K. A., Malloy, H. T. (1938) *J. Biol. Chem.* 126, 655.

Gartler, S. M. (1962) *at the* American Society of Human Genetics, Corv
     Oregon.
   — Gandini, E., Ceppellini, R. (1962) *Nature, Lond.* 193, 602.
Gorman, J. G., Dire, J., Treacy, A. M., Cahan, A. (1963) *J. Lab. Clin.*
     61, 642.
Harris, J. W. (1963) The Red Cell; p. 268. Cambridge, Mass.
Itano, H. A. (1950) PH.D. thesis for the California Institute of Technol.
Jacob, H. S., MacDonald, R. A., Jandl, J. H. (1962) *J. Clin. Invest.* 41,
Jalavisto, E., Solantera, L. (1959) *Acta Physiol. Scan.* 46, 274.
Jandl, J. H., Simmons, R. L., Castle, W. B. (1961) *Blood,* 268, 525.
Jung, F. (1949) *Dtsch. Arch. Klin. Med.* 195, 454.
Krill, A. E., Beutler, E. (1964) *Invest. Ophthal.* (in the press).
Lohr, G. W., Waller, H. D., Karges, O., Schlegel, B., Muller, A. A.
     Klin. Wschr. 36, 1008.
Lyon, M. F. (1961) *Nature, Lond.* 190, 372.
   — (1962) *Amer. J. Hum. Genet.* 14, 135.
Marks, P. A. (1958) *Science,* 127, 1338.
   — Gross, R. T. (1959) *J. Clin. Invest.* 38, 2253.
McKusick, V. A. (1962) *Ann. Int. Med.* 56, 991.
Motulsky, A. (1962) *at the* American Society of Human Genetics, Cor
     Oregon.
Ohno, S., Hauschka, T. S. (1960) *Cancer Res.* 20, 541.
   — Makino, S. (1961) *Lancet, i,* 78.
Pearson, C. M., Fowler, W. M., Wright, S. W. (1963) *Proc. Nat. Acad.*
     50, 24.
Reed, T. E., Simpson, N. E., Chown, B. (1963) *Lancet, ii,* 467.
Rundles, R. W., Falls, H. F. (1946) *Amer. J. Med. Sci.* 211, 641.

(From The Lancet, *January 25, 1964.)*

FURTHER READINGS

Ford, C. E., and Harris, H. (Eds.) New aspects of human genetics. *Br. Med. J.*
     25:1, 1969.
Giblett, E. R. *Genetic Markers in Human Blood.* Oxford: Blackwell, 1969.
Lerner, I. M. *Heredity, Evolution and Society.* San Francisco: Freeman, 1968.
McKusick, V. A. *Human Genetics* (2nd ed.). Englewood Cliffs, N. J.: Prentice-
     Hall, 1969.
McKusick, V. A. *Mendelian Inheritance in Men: Catalogs of Autosomal Domi-
     nant, Autosomal Recessive and X-linked Phenotypes.* Baltimore: Johns
     Hopkins, 1968.
Stern, C. *Principles of Human Genetics.* San Francisco: Freeman, 1960.

5 From Molecules to Information

STUDY GUIDE

The major objective of this unit is to understand how genetic information is stored and used. The short communication by Watson and Crick, reproduced here in its original, produced an avalanche of research that culminated in the deciphering of the genetic code and resulted in Nobel prizes in Biology and Medicine being given to a number of scientists in the last few years.

We will concentrate as much as possible on data obtained from mammalian cells, but quite a large part of the developments in this field come from bacteria and viruses. They are similar along general lines to *eukaryotic* (nucleus-containing) cells, but they also have a few special features.

After working through this chapter, you should be able to do the following:

1. Identify dividing cells and see the chromosomes in them, and describe the general features of and differences between mitosis and meiosis.

2. State the evidence for the localization of genetic information in chromosomes.

3. Describe the structure of ribonucleic and deoxyribonucleic acids, naming the hydrogen bases and sugars, and explain how they link to form nucleotides. Know the general structure of purines and pyrimidines.

4. State the evidence that genetic information is recorded in the structure of DNA, and explain its relation to chromosomal structure.

5. Understand, in the context of genetic information, the definitions of replication, transcription, and translation.

6. Describe the biochemical process for the replication of DNA and its translation to RNA.

7. Describe the role and structural peculiarities of different RNAs involved in the process of protein synthesis.

8. Describe the general features of the process of protein synthesis, and the points where some of its inhibitors act.

9. Describe the general features of the genetic code.

GENETIC INFORMATION

At the moment of conception, each individual receives from its parents a fantastic amount of information which leads to the growth and development of the egg, resulting in the complexity of the human body. The amount of information transmitted is inconceivably greater than the engineering specifications for even the most intricate machines.

As has been explained, living things express a large fraction of this required information by producing building blocks — proteins. Once synthesized, proteins assemble into their final configuration spontaneously, as we have seen with hemoglobin. Furthermore, protein molecules are capable of interacting with other molecules, or ions, to create a spontaneously organized tridimensional structure.

There are thousands of different proteins in the human body. Specifying just the amino acid composition is not enough. With the amino acids needed to build one chain of hemoglobin, it is possible to make about 10^{184} different sequences. The egg must be supplied with information about the exact sequence of amino acids for all the protein that the organism may produce.

Where and in what form is all this information stored such that it may be spread to all the cells of the body?

MITOSIS

With the use of time-lapse microphotography it is possible to record on film the whole process of cell division.

Study one of these films*, and compare it with actual slides of dividing cells from Ascaris, an intestinal parasite, to identify the steps schematized in Figure 5-1

**Mitosis in Animal Cells,* A. S. Bajer and A. F. Owczrazak, Harper and Row.

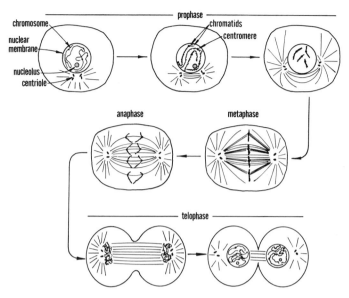

Fig. 5-1. Mitosis.

The most striking feature of cell division or *mitosis* (Fig. 5-1) is the progressive condensation of the chromosomes inside the nucleus. Each chromosome is made from two filaments called *chromatids,* which are linked by a *centromere.* As the nuclear membrane dissolves, the chromosomes are released into the cytoplasm. They order themselves about the cell's equator, and all the centromeres split in two simultaneously. Each chromatid is then pulled by aster fibers until it migrates to one of the poles of the cell. The chromosomes then uncoil, and two nuclei are formed. The cell divides, forming two new cells. The whole process takes about one hour.

The main part of the process is not visible under the microscope. About 15 hours before cell division begins with the condensation of the chromosomes, each chromatid must replicate so that during cell division one copy will migrate to each pole.

MEIOSIS

In 1833, Edouard van Beneden discovered that Ascaris cells have few chromosomes, which makes the process of cell division for the formation of sex cells (called *meiosis*) relatively simple to study in them. He observed that during the formation of the gametes, chromosomes do not replicate, with the result that cells have half the total number of chromosomes. When the egg and spermatozoon fuse together in fertilization, the regular number reappears, as each chromosome has a homologue, one contributed from the spermatozoon and the other from the egg.

Study a film showing cells undergoing meiosis*, and actual slides of Ascaris oocytes, and identify the steps schematized in Figure 5-2.

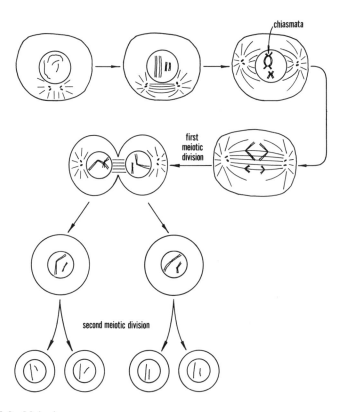

Fig. 5-2.   Meiosis.

Meiosis (Fig. 5-2) has been described down to its smallest details and, following the original description by Beneden, divided into a number of phases with complex names. Fundamentally, it starts like any mitosis, with chromosomes becoming visible by condensation, each showing its two chromatids.

*Meiosis, A. S. Bajer, Harper and Row.

Then each chromosome pairs lengthwise with its homologue. The pair begins to split apart so it is possible to see the two chromosomes linked by crossing points *(chiasmata)* as they separate. The nuclear membrane dissolves and the homologues part, migrating to the poles to form two nuclei. In contrast to a regular cell division, this results in chromosomes which are already duplicated. It is immediately followed by a second division in which, like the usual mitosis, the chromatids separate and migrate to opposite poles. These two special mitoses result in *haploid* cells, that is, cells with half the regular number of chromosomes for the species.

The parallel between Mendel's hypothetical hereditary factors, today called genes, and chromosomes was raised in a famous paper published in 1903 by Sutton. Each descendant receives half the chromosomes of each parent. For each pair of homologous chromosomes that he, in turn, passes on to each of his own descendants, he will transmit either the one received from his mother or the one received from his father. The potential number of different off-spring seems quite limited at first glance. Sutton calculated this number for species with different numbers of chromosomes, but stopped short at 36 (man has 46). When humans are considered, and one choice is selected from each pair of homologous chromosomes, it is found that one couple has the possibility of more than 70,000,000,000 different children!

CROSSING-OVER

At the turn of the century Morgan began to breed *Drosophila* (fruit flies), and in a paper published in 1910 he showed that white eye gene transmission is linked to sex determination. Goldschmidt related chromosomes to sex determination. The year after, Morgan showed that *Drosophila* genes are transmitted as if *linked* in four groups corresponding to the four chromosomes this species has. To a limited extent this linkage may be broken, separating genes that were originally linked on a specific chromosome. Morgan proposed that genes are linearly arranged on chromosomes, and that segregation results from an exchange of parts of homologous chromosomes during pairing in meiosis (seen as the chiasmata) (Fig. 5-3).

Fig. 5-3. Crossing-over.

In 1913, Sturtevand took Morgan's idea one step further. He calculated the percentage of recombinations of different genes on one chromosome. The farther apart two genes are, the greater the chance of their being separated by *crossing-over,* the genetic break that results in the chiasmata. So the frequency of recombination provides an indirect measure of distance and allows the construction of a genetic map. He found the genetic distance between A and B and between A and C (Fig. 5-4), and calculated the expected recombination frequency between B and C. This agreed quite well with experimental findings.

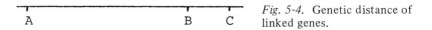

A	B	C

Fig. 5-4. Genetic distance of linked genes.

Drosophila have very large chromosomes in their salivary glands, which present a number of bands that may be stained with orcein. A detailed cytological map may be made for each chromosome. By comparing genetic maps with cytological maps, especially in many chromosome aberrations (as when parts are deleted or inverted), a correlation between genetic and actual distances in the salivary chromosomes and chromosomes of other cells is possible (Fig. 5-5). There is no simple correlation, as if condensation of the chromosome is not uniform and not all regions contain the same amount of genetic material.

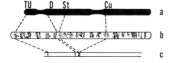

Fig. 5-5. Relationship of actual cytological distance in gonadal chromosomes (a) and salivary chromosomes (b) to the genetic map (c).

CHEMICAL COMPOSITION OF GENETIC INFORMATION

In 1871 Miescher treated pus with diluted hydrochloric acid, isolating nuclei that he could recognize under the microscope. To free the nuclei completely from any cytoplasm, he used an extract of pig stomach tissue. He then extracted the nuclei with sodium hydroxide, obtaining "a soluble nuclein" which on analysis contained 13.47 to 13.97% nitrogen, 1.78 to 2.00% sulfur, and 5.76 to 5.96% P_2O_5. In his paper he concluded: "It seems likely to me that a whole family of such phosphorus-containing substances, differing somewhat from each other, will emerge which perhaps will deserve equal consideration with the proteins. A knowledge of the relation between nuclear materials, proteins, and their immediate products of metabolism will gradually help to raise the curtain which at present so completely veils the inner process of cellular growth."

As pus was not an easy material to obtain, Miescher turned to salmon sperm, isolating from the nuclein a protein called *protamine.* This work was continued by Kossel, who used other materials to discover another group of proteins that bind to nucleic acids: histones. On hydrolyzing nucleic acids, he identified two groups of nitrogen-containing compounds: *purines* and *pyrimidines* (Fig. 5-6).

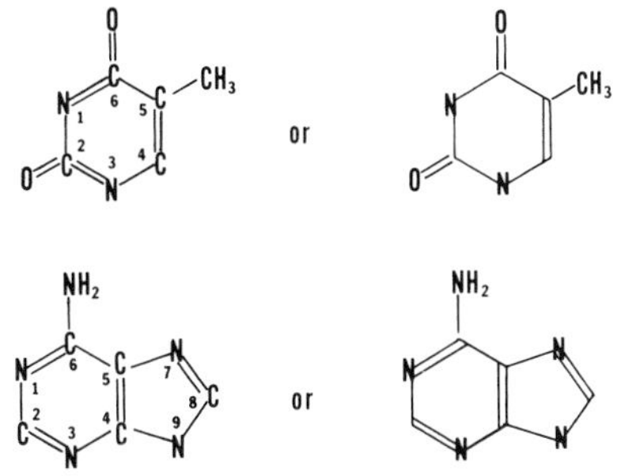

Fig. 5-6. Structure of pyrimidines (top) and purines (bottom).

In the first quarter of this century, studies concentrated on two nucleic acids. One was isolated from yeast and contained D-ribose, hence the name *ribonucleic acid.* The other was isolated from the thymus (a gland inside the chest on the back of the sternal bone) and was called *thymonucleic acid.* Both contained four basic components: phosphoric acid, a five-carbon sugar, purines, and pyrimidines. There were two differences, however: in the ribonucleic acid, the sugar is ribose; in the other acid, 2-deoxyribose (Fig. 5-7). Ribonucleic

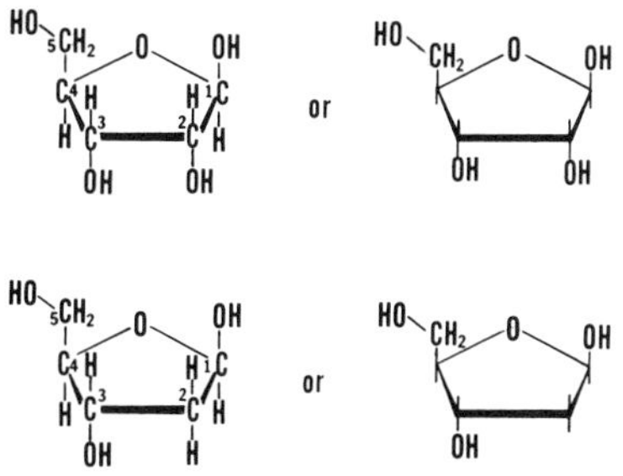

Fig. 5-7. Pentoses present in nucleic acids. Top, ribose; bottom, 2-deoxyribose

acid contains cytosine and uracil as pyrimidines; the other acid, thymine and cytosine (Fig. 5-8). Today the deoxyribose-containing nucleic acid is called *deoxyribonucleic acid* or *DNA,* and ribonucleic acid is referred to as *RNA.*

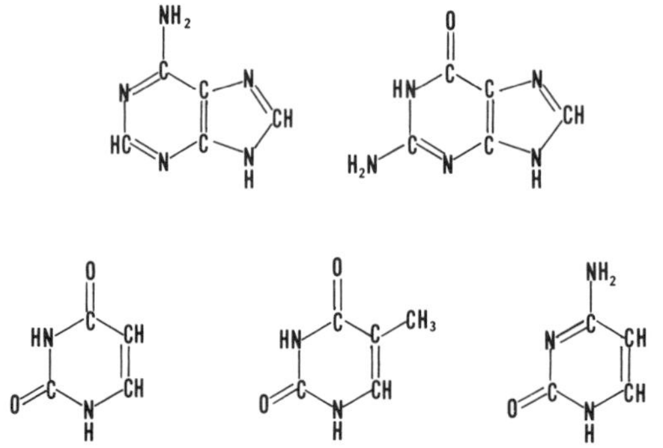

Fig. 5-8. Purines and pyrimidines in nucleic acids. Top, adenine and guanine; bottom, uracil, thymine, and cytosine.

In 1924, Feulgen developed a very important histochemical method for detecting DNA. DNA, but not RNA, hydrolyzes in a mild acid solution. This frees the aldehyde group of the pentose to react with reduced fuchsin. The reoxidized red fuchsin is bound as an insoluble complex that shows the distribution of DNA in cytological preparations. DNA was shown to exist in all nuclei in yeast, plants, and animal cells.

The structure of nucleic acids was established by degradation. DNA hydrolyzes in weak acid, liberating all purines and leaving behind an apurinic acid. RNA hydrolyzes in weak alkali, producing nucleotides with a pentose base and phosphoric acids (Fig. 5-9).

By chromatography of RNA which had been subjected to alkaline hydrolysis, eight nucleotides were found instead of the expected four (two adenylic acids, two uridylic acids, two guanylic acids, and two cytidylic acids). It was shown that each existed as a $2'$ and a $3'$ nucleotide. This led to some confusion until it was shown that the product of hydrolysis is a $2'-3'$ cyclic nucleotide that breaks to produce $2'$ and $3'$ nucleotide mixtures (Fig. 5-10).

A number of enzymes were used — some that break phosphodiester bonds and some specific for DNA or RNA, obtained from snake venom, the spleen, or the pancreas — that split the nucleic acid into either $5'$ or $3'$ nucleotides. This led to the structure shown in Figure 5-11, with diester phosphate bonds between the $3'$ position of one pentose and the $5'$ position of the next (the $3'$ notation is used so as not to be confused with the 3 position of the base).

There seemed to be little doubt that genetic information was stored in the nucleus. A striking experiment was conducted in 1943 by Hammerling, using *Acetabularia,* a seaweed (alga) that measures a few millimeters in length and is a single cell. *Acetabularia* looks like a small plant having a base (containing the nucleus), a stalk, and a cap. If it is cut into pieces, only the base survives. It is possible to transplant or graft the stalk of another species onto the base

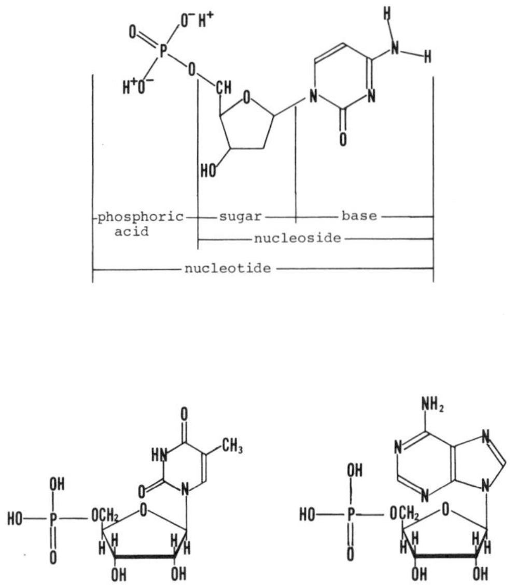

Fig. 5-9. Nucleotides. Top, general structure; bottom, a pyrimidine (Thymidine-5'-phosphate [TMP], Thymidylic acid [deoxi]) and a purine nucleotide (Adenosine-5'-phosphate [AMP] Adenylic acid).

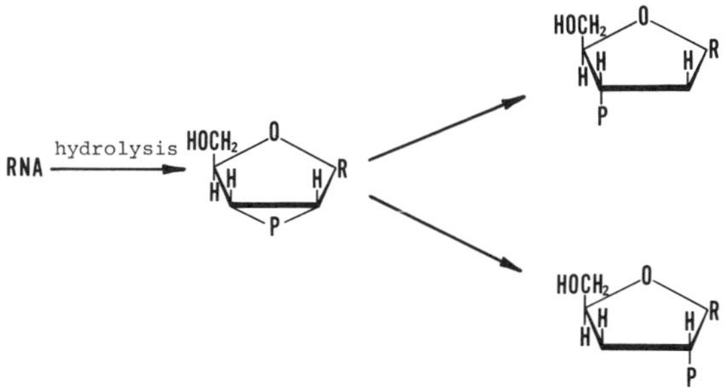

Fig. 5-10. Alkaline hydrolysis of RNA.

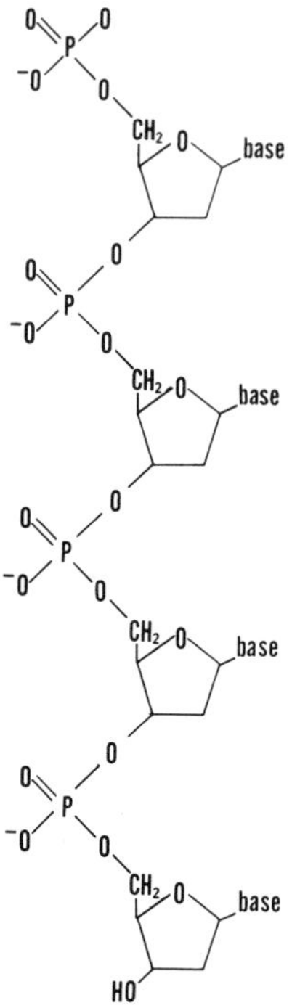

Fig. 5-11. Nucleic acid.

(Fig. 5-12). When the cap reforms on top of the grafted cell, it does so in the *Acetabularia* shape — that is, it is governed by the cell that provided the nucleus.

What type of molecule could store the very large amount of genetic information any individual carries? This problem was a major challenge until the fifties. The possible candidates did not look very promising: nucleic acids, protamines, and histones.

Nucleic acid seemed to be a very monotonous macromolecule with four building blocks. In the 1930s and 1940s, it was believed that this macromolecule was like any of the present artificial polymers used to make fibers — a long repetition of smaller units. It was even postulated that the smallest unit would have four nucleotides with a uniform sequence of the four nitrogen bases. (One of the ideas at that time was that proteins would have a similar structure — if a protein had 100 amino acids, 10 being proline, proline should appear regularly each tenth amino acid.)

Protamines are very small molecules, although they contain more building blocks than nucleic acids do (arginine, leucine, valine, alanine, glycine, proline, and serine). Each molecule has 27 amino acids, 19 being arginine. Histones are larger, with 180 amino acids, including most kinds of amino acids with the

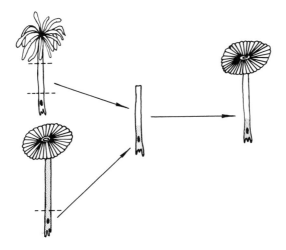

Fig. 5-12. Transplant of stalk part of *Acetabularia.*

notable exception of tryptophan. There are several types of histones, some
arginine-rich, others lysine-rich. The presence of the basic amino acids lysine
and arginine explains why protamines and histones combine with nucleic acids,
which are negatively charged.

Until the middle of the fifties, there were papers suggesting that histones and
protamines could carry genetic information. Of course, there are in the nucleus
other proteins with a more complex primary structure, some with phosphate
groups attached to the serine hydroxyl group (phosphoproteins), that could
be strong candidates for storing genetic information.

There are two ways of storing information. It can be recorded in a very
stable form that remains available for retrieval for a very long time, or it can
be stored in a not-so-stable form but recopied continuously so that it is never
lost. Recopying provides a slight chance each time of introducing error. After
the Second World War, radioactive phosphorus became available. By measuring the turnover of phosphorus compounds in vivo, Hevesy discovered, in 1946,
that RNA has a higher turnover than DNA. Other phosphorus-containing
compounds, like phospholipids and phosphoproteins, have even higher turn-
overs.

The distribution of DNA and RNA in the cell can be studied with proper
techniques. Both nucleic acids absorb intensively at 260 mμ and therefore
can be located with an ultraviolet microscope. RNA or DNA can be removed
from the preparation by the use of RNAse or DNAse, enzymes that digest just

one type of nucleic acid. Feulgen reagent is specific for DNA. Another histo-chemical staining process utilizes methyl green and pyronine, the first staining DNA in green, the second RNA in red. These methods can be quantified through the use of microspectrophotometers which measure the absorption in one small region under the microscope.

Whereas RNA is present both in the nucleus and in the cytoplasm, DNA was restricted to the nucleus. Using biochemical and microscopic methods, Boivin, Vendredy, and Vendredy showed in 1948 that different cells of the same species contained a constant amount of DNA (in some tissues four or eight times) and half this amount in the gametes.

In 1944, a very decisive experiment was carried out with bacteria. In 1928, Griffith had isolated two strains of pneumococcus. One grew in smooth colonies (and was called S strain), was very virulent, and showed a thick capsule under the microscope. The other, which grew in small, rough-looking colonies (R strain) without capsules, was not virulent. Griffith injected rats with R-strain together with heat-killed S-strain pneumococcus. The rats died, and from their blood he isolated S pneumococcus. A few years later, not only was this finding con-firmed, but it was shown that the transformation of R strain by S dead bacteria could occur in the test tube. R strain was cultivated in the presence of S-strain heat-killed pneumococcus and anti-R serum. The anti-R serum (from an animal immunized with R strain) agglutinated and killed R pneumococcus, so that only those organisms transformed into S grew. Then in 1944, Avery, McLeon, and McCarty isolated from heat-killed S pneumococcus a fraction that could trans-form R strain in culture, and showed that the activity was due to DNA.

Further proof came much later from a virus showing that nucleic acid was the only compound that entered a host cell and made the cell produce more virus.

THE WATSON-CRICK MODEL

In 1950, Chargaff analyzed the base composition of DNA in different species from yeast to men and found a remarkable regularity: the ratio of adenine to thymine (A/T) and guanine to cytosine (G/C) was 1. The different DNAs varied in the ratio A+T/G+C.

Chargaff's findings restricted even further the possible DNA structures. Meanwhile, the methods used to isolate DNA were improved. Keeping the molecule intact is a delicate matter because as soon as the cell structure is broken, DNA is exposed to a number of enzymes that hydrolyze the molecule (DNAses, phosphatases). Moreover, very long molecules are very fragile and break by shearing, not being able to support their own great weight in stress situations. With care, however, molecules of DNA with legths of 17 to 1,000 μ and molecular weights of 34 to 2,000 million were isolated from several sources. Since these molecules have from 10^5 to 10^7 nucleotides, recording an enormous amount of information on them presents no problem, even given that there are only four bases to use (guanine, cytosine, thymine, adenine), in pairs of A–T and G–C.

Pauling, who made brilliant contributions to solving the alpha helix structure of proteins, became interested in nucleic acids. In Cambridge, Wilkins concentrated on x-ray diffraction studies of nucleic acids. Two young researchers, Watson and Crick, devised a fantastic hypothesis which is summarized in the following two papers.

MOLECULAR STRUCTURE OF NUCLEIC ACIDS
A STRUCTURE FOR DEOXYRIBOSE NUCLEIC ACID

J. D. Watson, F. H. C. Crick

Medical Research Council Unit for the Study of the Molecular Structure of Biological Systems, Cavendish Laboratory, Cambridge. April 2.

We wish to suggest a structure for the salt of deoxyribose nucleic acid (D.N.A.). This structure has novel features which are of considerable biological interest.

A structure for nucleic acid has already been proposed by Pauling and Corey[1]. They kindly made their manuscript available to us in advance of publication. Their model consists of three intertwined chains, with the phosphates near the fibre axis, and the bases on the outside. In our opinion, this structure is unsatisfactory for two reasons: (1) We believe that the material which gives the X-ray diagrams is the salt, not the free acid. Without the acidic hydrogen atoms it is not clear what forces would hold the structure together, especially as the negatively charged phosphates near the axis will repel each other. (2) Some of the van der Waals distances appear to be too small.

Another three-chain structure has also been suggested by Fraser (in the press). In his model the phosphates are on the outside and the bases on the inside, linked together by hydrogen bonds. This structure as described is rather ill-defined, and for this reason we shall not comment on it.

We wish to put forward a radically different structure for the salt of deoxyribose nucleic acid. This structure has two helical chains each coiled round the same axis (see diagram). We have made the usual chemical assumptions, namely, that each chain consists of phosphate di-ester groups joining β-D-deoxyribofuranose residues with $3',5'$ linkages. The two chains (but not their bases) are related by a dyad

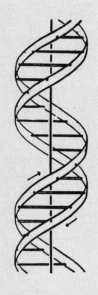

This figure is purely diagrammatic. The two ribbons symbolize the two phosphate-sugar chains, and the horizontal rods the pairs of bases holding the chains together. The vertical line marks the fibre axis

perpendicular to the fibre axis. Both chains follow right-handed helices, but owing to the dyad the sequences of the atoms in the two chains run in opposite directions. Each chain loosely resembles Furberg's[2] model No. 1; that is, the bases are on the inside of the helix and the phosphates on the outside. The configuration of the sugar and the atoms near it is close to Furberg's 'standard configuration', the sugar being roughly perpendicular to the attached base. There is a residue on each chain every 3.4 A. in the z-direction. We have assumed an angle of $36°$ between adjacent residues in the same chain, so that the structure repeats after 10 residues on each chain, that is, after 34 A. The distance of a phosphorus atom from the fibre axis is 10 A. As the phosphates are on the outside, cations have easy access to them.

The structure is an open one, and its water content is rather high. At lower water contents we would expect the bases to tilt so that the structure could become more compact.

The novel feature of the structure is the manner in which the two chains are held together by the purine and pyrimidine bases. The planes of the bases are perpendicular to the fibre axis. They are joined together in pairs, a single base from one chain being hydrogen-bonded to a single base from the other chain, so that the two lie side by side with identical z-co-ordinates. One of the pair must be a purine and the other a pyrimidine for bonding to occur. The hydrogen bonds are made as follows: purine position 1 to pyrimidine position 1; purine position 6 to pyrimidine position 6.

If it is assumed that the bases only occur in the structure in the most plausible tautomeric forms (that is, with the keto rather than the enol configurations) it is found that only specific pairs of bases can bond together. These pairs are: adenine (purine) with thymine (pyrimidine), and guanine (purine) with cytosine (pyrimidine).

In other words, if an adenine forms one member of a pair, on either chain, then on these assumptions the other member must be thymine; similarly for guanine and cytosine. The sequence of bases on a single chain does not appear to be restricted in any way. However, if only specific pairs of bases can be formed, it follows that if the sequence of bases on one chain is given, then the sequence on the other chain is automatically determined.

It has been found experimentally[3,4] that the ratio of the amounts of adenine to thymine, and the ratio of guanine to cytosine, are always very close to unity for deoxyribose nucleic acid.

It is probably impossible to build this structure with a ribose sugar in place of the deoxyribose, as the extra oxygen atom would make too close a van der Waals contact.

The previously published X-ray data[5,6] on deoxyribose nucleic acid are insufficient for a rigorous test of our structure. So far as we can tell, it is roughly compatible with the experimental data, but it must be regarded as unproved until it has been checked against more exact results. Some of these are given in the following communications. We were not aware of the details of the results presented there when we devised our structure, which rests mainly though not entirely on published experimental data and stereochemical arguments.

It has not escaped our notice that the specific pairing we have postulated immediately suggests a possible copying mechanism for the genetic material.

Full details of the structure, including the conditions assumed in building it, together with a set of co-ordinates for the atoms, will be published elsewhere.

We are much indebted to Dr. Jerry Donohue for constant advice and criticism, especially on interatomic distances. We have also been stimulated by a knowledge of the general nature of the unpublished experimental results and ideas of Dr. M. H. F. Wilkins, Dr. R. E. Franklin and their co-workers at King's College, London. One of us (J. D. W.) has been aided by a fellowship from the National Foundation for Infantile Paralysis.

[1]Pauling, L., and Corey, R. B., *Nature*, 171, 346 (1953); *Proc. U.S. Nat. Acad. Sci.*, 39, 84 (1953).
[2]Furberg, S., *Acta Chem. Scand.*, 6, 634 (1952).
[3]Chargaff, E., for references see Zamenhof, S., Brawerman, G., and Chargaff, E., *Biochim. et Biophys. Acta*, 9, 402 (1952).
[4]Wyatt, G. R., *J. Gen. Physiol.*, 36, 201 (1952).
[5]Astbury, W. T., Symp. Soc. Exp. Biol. 1, Nucleic Acid. 66 (Camb. Univ. Press, 1947).
[6]Wilkins, M. H. F., and Randall, J. T., *Biochim. et Biophys. Acta*, 10, 192 (1953).

GENETICAL IMPLICATIONS OF THE STRUCTURE OF DEOXYRIBONUCLEIC ACID

J. D. Watson, F. H. C. Crick

Medical Research Council Unit for the Study of the Molecular Structure of Biological Systems, Cavendish Laboratory, Cambridge

The importance of deoxyribonucleic acid (DNA) within living cells is undisputed. It is found in all dividing cells, largely if not entirely in the nucleus, where it is an essential constituent of the chromosomes. Many lines of evidence indicate that it is the carrier of a part of (if not all) the genetic specificity of the chromosomes and thus of the gene itself. Until now, however, no evidence has been presented to show how it might carry out the essential operation required of a genetic material, that of exact self-duplication.

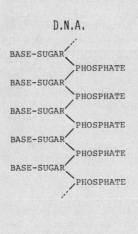

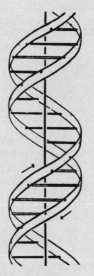

Fig. 1. Chemical formula of a single chain of deoxyribonucleic acid.

Fig. 2. This figure is purely diagrammatic. The two ribbons symbolize the two phosphate-sugar chains, and the horizontal rods the pairs of bases holding the chains together. The vertical line marks the fibre axis.

1

2

We have recently proposed a structure[1] for the salt of deoxyribonucleic acid which, if correct, immediately suggests a mechanism for its self-duplication. X-ray evidence obtained by the workers at King's College, London[2], and presented at the same time, gives qualitative support to our structure and is incompatible with all previously proposed structures[3]. Though the structure will not be completely proved until a more extensive comparison has been made with the X-ray data, we now feel sufficient confidence in its general correctness to discuss its genetical implications. In doing so we are assuming that fibres of the salt of deoxyribonucleic acid are not artefacts arising in the method of preparation, since it has been shown by Wilkins and his co-workers that similar

X-ray patterns are obtained from both the isolated fibres and certain intact biological materials such as sperm head and bacteriophage particles[3,4].

The chemical formula of deoxyribonucleic acid is now well established. The molecule is a very long chain, the backbone of which consists of a regular alternation of sugar and phosphate groups, as shown in Fig. 1. To each sugar is attached a nitrogenous base, which can be of four different types. (We have considered 5-methyl cytosine to be equivalent to cytosine, since either can fit equally well into our structure.) Two of the possible bases—adenine and guanine—are purines, and the other two—thymine and cytosine—are pyrimidines. So far as is known, the sequence of bases along the chain is irregular. The monomer unit, consisting of phosphate, sugar and base, is known as a nucleotide.

The first feature of our structure which is of biological interest is that it consists not of one chain, but of two. These two chains are both coiled around a common fibre axis, as is shown diagrammatically in Fig. 2. It has often been assumed that since there was only one chain in the chemical formula there would only be one in the structural unit. However, the density, taken with the X-ray evidence[2], suggests very strongly that there are two.

The other biologically important feature is the manner in which the two chains are held together. This is done by hydrogen bonds between the bases, as shown schematically in Fig. 3. The bases are joined

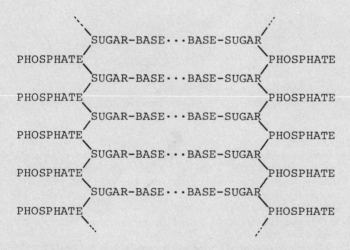

Fig. 3. Chemical formula of a pair of deoxyribonucleic acid chains. The hydrogen bonding is symbolized by dotted lines.

together in pairs, a single base from one chain being hydrogen-bonded to a single base from the other. The important point is that only certain pairs of bases will fit into the structure. One member of a pair must be a purine and the other a pyrimidine in order to bridge between the two chains. If a pair consisted of two purines, for example, there would not be room for it.

We believe that the bases will be present almost entirely in their most probable tautomeric forms. If this is true, the conditions for forming hydrogen bonds are more restrictive, and the only pairs of bases possible are:

adenine with thymine;

guanine with cytosine.

The way in which these are joined together is shown in Figs. 4 and 5. A given pair can be either way round. Adenine, for example, can occur on either chain; but when it does, its partner on the other chain must always be thymine.

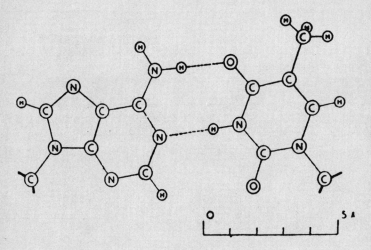

Fig. 4. Pairing of adenine (left) and thymine (right). Hydrogen bonds are shown dotted. One carbon atom of each sugar is shown.

This pairing is strongly supported by the recent analytical results[5], which show that for all sources of deoxyribonucleic acid examined the amount of adenine is close to the amount of thymine, and the amount of guanine close to the amount of cytosine, although the cross-ratio (the ratio of adenine to guanine) can vary from one source to another. Indeed, if the sequence of bases on one chain is irregular, it is difficult to explain these analytical results except by the sort of pairing we have suggested.

The phosphate-sugar backbone of our model is completely regular, but any sequence of the pairs of bases can fit into the structure. It follows that in a long molecule many different permutations are possible, and it therefore seems likely that the precise sequence of the bases is the code which carries the genetical information. If the actual order of the bases on one of the pair of chains were given, one could write down the exact order of the bases on the other one, because of the specific pairing. Thus, one chain is, as it were, the complement of the other, and it is this

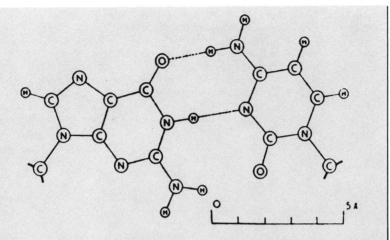

Fig. 5. Pairing of guanine (left) and cytosine (right). Hydrogen bonds are shown dotted. One carbon atom of each sugar is shown.

feature which suggests how the deoxyribonucleic acid molecule might duplicate itself.

Previous discussions of self-duplication have usually involved the concept of a template, or mould. Either the template was supposed to copy itself directly or it was to produce a 'negative', which in its turn was to act as a template and produce the original 'positive' once again. In no case has it been explained in detail how it would do this in terms of atoms and molecules.

Now our model for deoxyribonucleic acid is, in effect, a *pair* of templates, each of which is complementary to the other. We imagine that prior to duplication the hydrogen bonds are broken, and the two chains unwind and separate. Each chain then acts as a template for the formation on to itself of a new companion chain, so that eventually we shall have *two* pairs of chains, where we only had one before. Moreover, the sequence of the pairs of bases will have been duplicated exactly.

A study of our model suggests that this duplication could be done most simply if the single chain (or the relevant portion of it) takes up the helical configuration. We imagine that at this stage in the life of the cell, free nucleotides, strictly polynucleotide precursors, are available in quantity. From time to time the base of a free nucleotide will join up by hydrogen bonds to one of the bases on the chain already formed. We now postulate that the polymerization of these monomers to form a new chain is only possible if the resulting chain can form the proposed structure. This is plausible, because steric reasons would not allow nucleotides 'crystallized' on to the first chain to approach one another in such a way that they could be joined together into a new chain, unless they were those nucleotides which were necessary to form our structure. Whether a special enzyme is required to carry out the polymerization, or whether the single helical chain already formed acts effectively as an enzyme, remains to be seen.

Since the two chains in our model are intertwined it is essential for them to untwist if they are to separate. As they make one complete turn around each other in 34 A., there will be about 150 turns per million molecular weight, so that whatever the precise structure of the chromosome a considerable amount of uncoiling would be necessary. It is well known from microscopic observation that much coiling and uncoiling occurs during mitosis, and though this is on a much larger scale it probably reflects similar processes on a molecular level. Although it is difficult at the moment to see how these processes occur without everything getting tangled, we do not feel that this objection will be insuperable.

Our structure, as described[1], is an open one. There is room between the pair of polynucleotide chains (see Fig. 2) for a polypeptide chain to wind around the same helical axis. It may be significant that the distance between adjacent phosphorus atoms, 7.1 A., is close to the repeat of a fully extended polypeptide chain. We think it probable that in the sperm head, and in artificial nucleoproteins, the polypeptide chain occupies this position. The relative weakness of the second layer-line in the published X-ray pictures[3a,4] is crudely compatible with such an idea. The function of the protein might well be to control the coiling and uncoiling, to assist in holding a single polynucleotide chain in a helical configuration, or some other non-specific function.

Our model suggests possible explanations for a number of other phenomena. For example, spontaneous mutation may be due to a base occasionally occurring in one of its less likely tautomeric forms. Again, the pairing between homologous chromosomes at meiosis may depend on pairing between specific bases. We shall discuss these ideas in detail elsewhere.

For the moment, the general scheme we have proposed for the reproduction of deoxyribonucleic acid must be regarded as speculative. Even if it is correct, it is clear from what we have said that much remains to be discovered before the picture of genetic duplication can be described in detail. What are the polynucleotide precursors? What makes the pair of chains unwind and separate? What is the precise role of the protein? Is the chromosome one long pair of deoxyribonucleic acid chains, or does it consist of patches of the acid joined together by protein?

Despite these uncertainties we feel that our proposed structure for deoxyribonucleic acid may help to solve one of the fundamental biological problems—the molecular basis of the template needed for genetic replication. The hypothesis we are suggesting is that the template is the pattern of bases formed by one chain of the deoxyribonucleic acid and that the gene contains a complementary pair of such templates.

One of us (J. D. W.) has been aided by a fellowship from the National Foundation for Infantile Paralysis (U.S.A.).

[1]Watson, J. D., and Crick, F. H. C., *Nature,* 171, 737 (1953).
[2]Wilkins, M. H. F., Stokes, A. R., and Wilson, M. R., *Nature,* 171, 738 (1953). Franklin, R. E., and Gosling, R. G., *Nature,* 171, 740 (1953).
[3](a) Astbury, W. T., Symp. No. 1 Soc. Exp. Biol., 66 (1947). (b) Furberg, S., *Acta Chem. Scand.,* 6, 634 (1952). (c) Pauling, L., and Corey, R. B., *Nature,* 171, 346 (1953); *Proc. U.S. Nat. Acad. Sci.,* 39, 84 (1953). (d) Fraser, R. D. B. (in preparation).
[4]Wilkins, M. H. F., and Randall, J. T., *Biochim. et Biophys. Acta,* 10, 192 (1953).
[5]Chargaff, E., for references see Zamenhof, S., Brawerman, G., and Chargaff, E., *Biochim. et Biophys. Acta,* 9, 402 (1952). Wyatt, G. R., *J. Gen. Physiol.* 36, 201 (1952).

Questions

1. If cells are cultivated in a medium containing tritium-labeled thymidine until they divide once, part of the DNA (that which is newly synthesized) will contain the ³H label. Now, if the cells are transferred to a regular medium for another cycle, so that each initial cell results in four cells, which one of the schemes shown in Figure 5-13 would be expected from the Watson-Crick model?

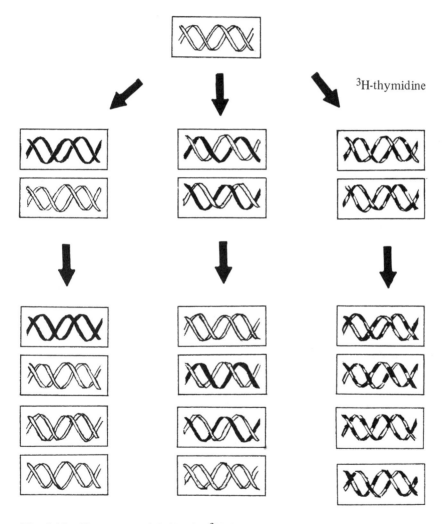

³H-thymidine

Fig. 5-13. Chromosome labeling by ³H-thymidine pulse during successive cell divisions.

2. Examine the autoradiograph in Figure 5-14. What conclusions can be drawn from it?

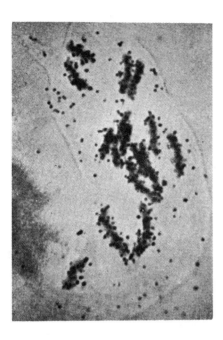

Fig. 5-14. Autoradiograph of a chromosome of a root-tip cell after one duplication in ³H-thymidine. Further division is blocked by colchicine. (Courtesy of J. H. Taylor, *Proc. X Int. Cong. Genet.,* 1958.)

3. In a companion paper published in the same issue of Nature, *Wilkins and his co-workers reported on their x-ray diffraction studies of purified DNA from E. coli, sperm heads, bacterial viruses, and pneumococcus-transforming principle. Their data agreed with Watson and Crick's proposed structure.*

Make a list of the biological implications of the Watson-Crick model, based on the preceding papers. Point out difficulties, and present ideas for experiments that could test this model.

An important experiment using lily root tips was carried out by Taylor in 1957–1958. He labeled newly produced DNA with ³H-thymidine, returning the roots to the regular medium so that the thymidine was available for only one cell division. The distribution of the isotope was detected by autoradiography (Fig. 5-15).

In Taylor's experiment, all the chromosomes were labeled on the first mitosis and half in the second, as predicted by Watson and Crick's semiconservative model. Part of the chromosomes have regions attached to ³H-thymidine and part are unlabeled, as if they have undergone an exchange similar to a

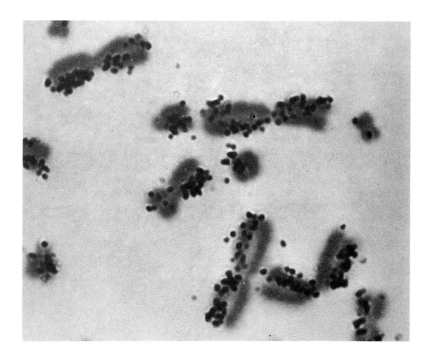

Fig. 5-15. Chromosomes labeled with ³H-thymidine. (Courtesy of G. Marin and D. M. Prescott, *J. Cell Biol.* 21:159, 1969.)

cross-over. As this is mitosis and not meiosis, the interpretation is that, after replication, there is a four-stranded break and exchange. This exchange occurs between two identical chromosomes so it does not lead to any genetic consequences, but it is visible in Taylor's experiment. He called this a *sister exchange*. For a single four-stranded break, the exchanges in Figure 5-16 may be expected.

The Watson-Crick DNA model assumes that the two strands have opposing polarity and are complementary, so that A pairs with T, and G with C (Fig. 5-17). If we assume that a chromosome is a single DNA molecule, part of the exchanges in Figure 5-17 are impossible, if exchange can occur only between chains with the same polarity. (Can you cross out the ones for which this is true?) Studying double sister exchanges, Taylor calculated the proper proportions to support the idea that chromosomes are made by a single DNA molecule. Similar results were obtained with human white cell chromosomes.

LABORATORY INVESTIGATION: PROPERTIES OF DNA

The properties of a preparation of DNA may be studied by two physical methods: ultraviolet absorption at 260 nm and viscosity. Investigate the effects of the following treatments:

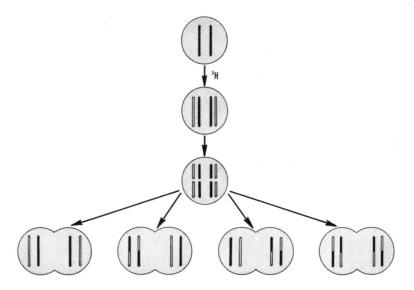

Fig. 5-16. The effect of sister exchanges as found in Taylor's experiment with ³H-thymidine-labeled chromosomes.

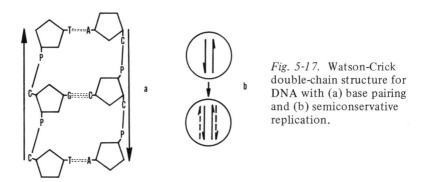

Fig. 5-17. Watson-Crick double-chain structure for DNA with (a) base pairing and (b) semiconservative replication.

1. Dilute several 0.1 ml samples of DNA solution to 4.0 ml with distilled water. Add various amounts of acid or base to achieve different pH's between 2.0 and 12.5. Complete the volume to 5.0 ml with distilled water. Measure the optical density and viscosity of each sample. Neutralize the samples to see if the effects are reversible.

2. Dilute a DNA sample ten times with 0.05M borate buffer at pH 8.5. Divide it into five samples and heat each for five minutes in a water bath at a different one of the following temperatures: 60, 70, 80, 90, and 100°C. Cool rapidly in an ice bath, and measure optical density and viscosity.

3. Dilute DNA ten times in SSC with $0.1M$ tris buffer, pH 7.5. Heat for five minutes at $100°C$, turn off the bath, and let cool very slowly to room temperature. Repeat in the presence of 2% formaldehyde. Measure optical density and viscosity.

4. Dilute DNA ten times with SSC containing $0.1M$ tris at pH 7.5 and $0.02M$ $MgCl_2$. Add 5 μg purified DNAse to the solution and incubate at room temperature. Follow the change in optical density at 260 nm. When it stabilizes, measure the viscosity.

5. Now investigate the kinetics of DNAse action on DNA by observing the change in viscosity during the enzymatic reaction. Measure the viscosity of the DNA solution, add the enzyme, and measure the viscosity at regular intervals of time thereafter.

Preparation of DNA

Use either ox thymus, obtained from a slaughterhouse and kept under ice, or fresh rat liver. Cut it into small pieces and homogenize 3 g in a Waring blender with 20 ml of $0.15M$ sodium chloride containing $0.1M$ edetic acid (EDTA) at a pH of 8.0. Filter through two layers of cheesecloth into a 250 ml flask; add, while stirring, 2 ml of 25% sodium docecyl sulfate (SDS); and place in a 60° water bath for 10 minutes. Cool at room temperature, and add 5 ml of $6M$ sodium perchloride while stirring gently. Add an equal volume of chloroform—isoamyl alcohol (24:1 v/v), stopper, and shake for 15 minutes. Remove the stopper every so often to release the pressure. Transfer to centrifuge tubes, and centrifuge at about 200 g for 10 minutes.

Carefully transfer the upper aqueous layer to another flask, and gently add a layer of 70 ml of ethanol over the solution. Mix very gently with the stirring rod. DNA will spool on the rod. Squeeze out the excess liquid.

Dissolve the spooled DNA in 10 ml of water and 1 ml of NaCl-EDTA. It may need to sit overnight. Add 0.5 ml SDS and then 2 ml 6 N sodium perchloride. Add 15 ml chloroform—isoamyl alcohol and shake. Remove the aqueous solution and precipitate as before with ethanol, spool the DNA, and dissolve it in $0.1 \times$ SSC ($0.15M$ NaCl and $0.015M$ sodium citrate diluted ten times to make $0.1 \times$ SSC). Add ten volumes of $1 \times$ SSC and let it dissolve, stirring very gently.

This preparation may be further purified by adding isopropanol under constant gentle stirring until it abruptly precipitates. The DNA is then dissolved as before.

Measurement by Ultraviolet Absorption

Proteins and nucleic acids absorb ultraviolet light at 260 nm. At 280 nm the absorption is mainly due to protein. Warburg established a method of measuring the approximate amount of proteins and nucleic acid from the 260 and 280 nm absorptions.

Calculate the amount of nucleic acids and proteins in your DNA sample, using the nomogram in Figure 5-18. Dilute the preparation with SSC containing 0.1M tris, pH 7.0, so that it gives an optical density at 260 nm of 0.5 when diluted 1:10. Keep it at 4.0°C.

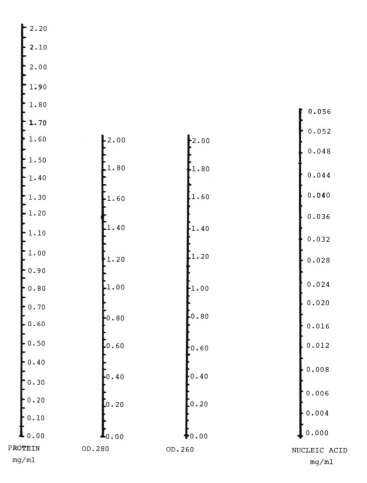

Fig. 5-18. Nomogram for calculating nucleic acid and protein concentration in a solution by ultraviolet absorption.

Measurement of Viscosity

Relative viscosity is measured by comparing the flow of solvent and solution through a narrow tube. This is done in a simple glass device called an *Ostwald viscosimeter* (Fig. 5-19). As viscosity varies with temperature, the viscosimeter is held in a water bath at a temperature regulated within ± 0.5°C. The solution

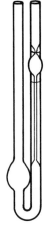

Fig. 5-19.   Viscosimeter.

is also equilibrated at the bath temperature. The liquid is then introduced into the viscosimeter, aspirated so that it goes above the upper mark, and allowed to flow down to the lower mark. The time taken to reach the lower mark is recorded for the pure solvent (t_0) and for the solution (t). The *viscosity* can be calculated by the formula

$$n = \frac{t - t_0}{Ct_0}$$

where C = concentration and n = viscosity.

If viscosity is measured at different concentrations, and n is plotted against C, the viscosity for zero concentration can be calculated. This is called the *intrinsic viscosity* (n_{C_0}).

The intrinsic viscosity for spherical particles is related to their diameter. For long molecules, the relation is more complex, but it is still related to size and shape and therefore to molecular weight. An empirical formula used to measure the molecular weight of DNA is

$$0.655 \log MW = 3.86 + \log (n_{C_0} + 0.5)$$

As in most experiments, you are comparing viscosities of samples of DNA which have been subjected to various treatments. The intrinsic viscosity need not be calculated to get a feel for how viscosity of DNA is affected by these various treatments; simply determine the ratio t/t_0 for each sample.

Measurement of DNAse Action on DNA

If DNA is a single long molecule, and DNAse acts by breaking bonds at random, the molecule will shorten, and viscosity decrease, in direct proportion to time. If DNA is double-stranded, viscosity will decrease only when both strands are hydrolyzed: therefore, viscosity will decrease with the square of time. If DNA is triple-stranded, viscosity will decrease proportionally to the cube of time.

$$1 - \frac{n_t}{n_0} = at^b$$

where n_0 = initial viscosity and n_t = viscosity at time t. Instead of viscosity, (n) the ratio between the flow time for the samples (t) and the solvent (t_0) can be used. Take the log:

$$\log \left(1 - \frac{n_t}{n_0} \right) = (\log a) + (b \log t)$$

Plot $\log (1 - \frac{n_t}{n_0})$ against $\log t$, and find out the strandedness of DNA.

DNA STRUCTURE AND REPLICATION

The result of the preceding experiments can be explained by the Watson-Crick model. The nitrogen bases are linked by hydrogen bonds. At high temperature or extreme pH, those bonds are broken, destroying the double helix and releasing the two strands.

More hydrogens become titratable and more are available for exchange with deuterium ions when heavy water is added to the solution. The rigid structure and long chains of DNA result in a very high viscosity that lessens when the double helix collapses or when the DNA chains are broken into smaller units. When different DNAs are compared, the "melting point" is found to be higher for the DNA with more GC pairs, which are bonded by three hydrogen bonds per pair as compared to two for the AT pair.

Due to the regular stacking of the nitrogen bases, particularly AT, double helix DNA absorbs less light at 260 nm than the random coil, or free nucleotides. When the double helix structure is destroyed, there is a hyperchromatic effect.

Ultracentrifugation

A very important tool for studying DNA and other macromolecules is ultracentrifugation. The material is spun in a high speed centrifuge that can reach centrifugal forces of 100,000 to 400,000 g. The macromolecules move down according to their size, shape, and density, opposed by the viscosity of the medium and by buoyancy. Analytical centrifuges are equipped with optical systems that permit continuous surveillance of the sedimentation. It is thus possible to determine whether the preparation is homogeneous or has other macromolecular components and, from the rate of sedimentation (and independent measurement of the diffusion constant), to calculate the molecular weight.

A very ingenious method was developed for studying macromolecules in the ultracentrifuge. Material is dissolved in $7.7M$ cesium chloride sediments, forming a linear gradient, with the top of the tube having a density of about 1.65 and the bottom about 1.76. Each macromolecule finds a point of equilibrium, collecting *(banding)* at that point of the gradient whose density equals its own. Very small differences can then be detected.

Meselson-Stahl Experiment

Meselson and Stahl, who developed this method, conducted a remarkable experiment in 1958. They grew *E. coli* bacteria for many generations in a medium containing ammonium chloride with ^{15}N as the source of nitrogen, so that the DNA was completely labeled with the heavy nitrogen. Then the culture was abruptly changed to normal ammonium chloride medium, with ^{14}N. DNA was isolated and submitted to the cesium chloride gradient centrifugation.

According to the Watson-Crick model, a hybrid ^{14}N–^{15}N DNA is expected in the first generation. In the second generation, equal amounts of ^{14}N and ^{14}N–^{15}N are expected. Study the original Meselson and Stahl illustrations (Figs. 5-20, 5-21). What do they show?

They also denatured the DNA preparations by heating, and submitted the sample to the cesium chloride gradient. As Figure 5-21 shows, the hybrid DNA is composed of two chains of different density, similar to a heated mixture of ^{15}N and ^{14}N DNA.

The Taylor experiment showed that the DNA chains distributed themselves according to the Watson-Crick model. The Meselson and Stahl experiment demonstrated that the chains replicated according to that model. A similar experiment was conducted with human white cells using bromouracil instead of uracil for labeling. The results supported the same conclusions.

LABORATORY INVESTIGATION: CHROMOSOMES

1. Put one drop of a growing culture of *Euplotes,* a free-living protozoon, on a microscope slide. Add one drop of 0.1% methyl green and one drop of $0.2M$ acetate buffer, pH 4.8. Cover with a cover slide.

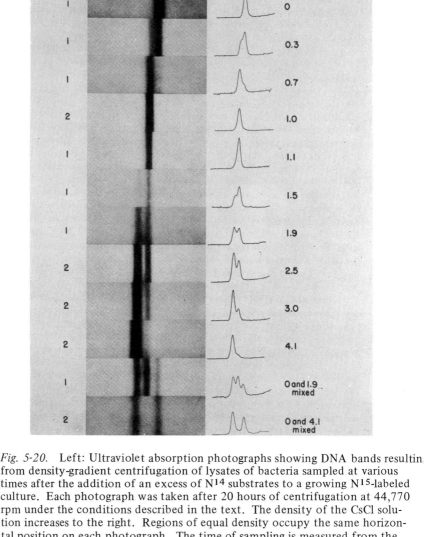

Fig. 5-20. Left: Ultraviolet absorption photographs showing DNA bands resultin from density-gradient centrifugation of lysates of bacteria sampled at various times after the addition of an excess of N^{14} substrates to a growing N^{15}-labeled culture. Each photograph was taken after 20 hours of centrifugation at 44,770 rpm under the conditions described in the text. The density of the CsCl solution increases to the right. Regions of equal density occupy the same horizontal position on each photograph. The time of sampling is measured from the time of the addition of N^{14} in units of the generation time. The generation times for Experiments 1 and 2 were estimated from measurements of bacterial growth Right: Microdensitometer tracings of the DNA bands shown in the adjacent photographs. The microdensitometer pen displacement above the base line is directly proportional to the concentration of DNA. The degree of labeling of a species of DNA corresponds to the relative position of its band between the bands of fully labeled and unlabeled DNA shown in the lowermost frame, which serves as a density reference. A test of the conclusion that the DNA in the band of intermediate density is just half-labeled is provided by the frame showing the mixture of generations 0 and 1.9. When allowance is made for the relative amounts of DNA in the three peaks, the peak of intermediate density is found to be centered at 50 ± 2 per cent of the distance between the N^{14} and N^{15} peaks.(Courtesy of M. Meselson and F. W. Stahl, *Proc. Nat. Acad. Sci.* 44:671, 1958.)

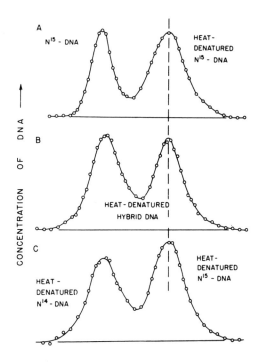

Fig. 5-21. The dissociation of the subunits of *E. coli* DNA upon heat denaturation. Each smooth curve connects points obtained by microdensitometry of an
ultraviolet absorption photograph taken after 20 hours of centrifugation in
CsCl solution at 44,770 rpm. The baseline density has been removed by subtraction. *A:* A mixture of heated and unheated N^{15} bacterial lysates. Heated
lysate alone gives one band in the position indicated. Unheated lysate was
added to this experiment for comparison. Heating has brought about a density
increase of 0.016 gm. cm.$^{-3}$ and a reduction of about half in the apparent
molecular weight of the DNA. *B:* Heated lysate of N^{15} bacteria grown for one
generation in N^{14} growth medium. Before heat denaturation, the hybrid DNA
contained in this lysate forms only one band, as may be seen in Fig. 5-4. *C:* A
mixture of heated N^{14} and heated N^{15} bacterial lysates. The density difference
is 0.015 gm. cm.$^{-3}$. (Courtesy of M. Meselson, and F. W. Stahl, *Proc. Nat.
Acad. Sci.* 44:671, 1958.)

Methyl green stains DNA. Observe several protozoa, make drawings of your observations, and describe any possible conclusions.

2. Examine a slide of human chromosomes.

DNA AND CHROMOSOMES

Our understanding of the structure of chromosomes has evolved from different fields and techniques of research and is still incomplete.

Early cytologists coined the word *chromatin* to describe a peculiar substance from which chromosomes were made. In the forties, Mirsky and Allfrey developed techniques for cell fractionation, obtaining intact nuclei and extracting several subfractions. Later, chromosomes could be isolated from cells arrested during mitosis. In the fifties, Casperson and Edstrom developed microspectrophotometric methods to analyze intracellular structure without breaking cells. More recently, electron microscopy has provided not only morphological data, but, by measurement of electron scattering, some chemical information.

Genetic experiments indicated that genes must remain linked and ordered throughout the cell cycle, including the period of interphase between cell divisions when chromosomes are not visible. Observing the appearance of chromosomes in the beginning of mitosis and the reconstitution of the sister nucleus at the end led to the suggestion that chromosomes must uncoil as a long, thin random fiber below the limits of visibility of the light microscope. Coiling was occasionally visible in some nuclei (Fig. 5-22).

Early electron microscopy did not show any intranuclear chromosomes. The best preparations, developed in the late sixties by DuPraw, showed the chromosomes and intact nuclear, trypsin-resistant fibers that dissolve when treated with DNAse and have a diameter of 23 nm. The chromosomes are made by densely packed and perhaps randomly coiled fibers.

The human cell nucleus contains 5.6 picograms (10^{-12} g) of DNA, which, according to the Watson-Crick model, would be 1740 mm long. This DNA is divided among 46 chromosomes, the longest of which measures about 10 μ and contains 0.23 picograms of DNA. The DNA in the longest chromosome, as an extended double helix, would measure 73 mm, or 73,000 μ. Electron microscopy shows 1,300 μ of the 23 nm fiber. The fiber is packed 56 times (1.300/73,000) and is folded another 130 times to fill the 10-μ chromosome.

Chromatin contains about 30 percent DNA, an equivalent percentage of histones, and 5 percent RNA, and the rest consists of other proteins. Equal weights of histone and DNA have equal numbers of basic amino and phosphate groups, which are linked by electrostatic charges. DNA and histone synthesis in the cell nucleus increase in parallel during DNA replication.

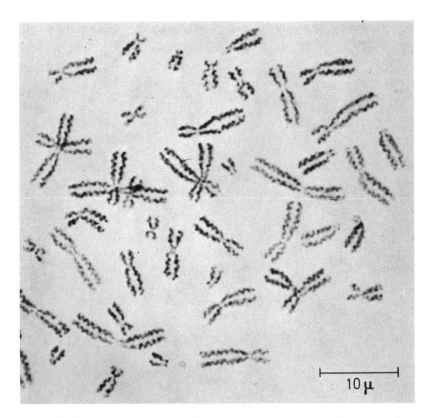

Fig. 5-22. Human chromosomes after hypotonic treatment. (Courtesy of Y. Ohnuki, *Nature* 208:916, 1965.)

The Coiling-Uncoiling Process

DNA is thus present as a supercoil bound to histones. By an unknown process, this coiling packs together during mitosis or meiosis and is released in the interphase. There does not seem to be a very simple, regular, coiled structure as one would imagine from the constant, definitive position of genes in cytological maps. This supercoiling must occur with some kind of regularity, however, although it looks very random. One proposed structure is the folded-fiber model of DuPraw (Fig. 5-23).

This brings us back to the uncoiling of the double helix, a necessary step for replication. In DuPraw's scheme, one sees the uncoiling starting at the ends and the uncoiling-duplication-recoiling process progressing to the center. This is apparently similar to the *Euplotes* DNA replication in the preceding laboratory,

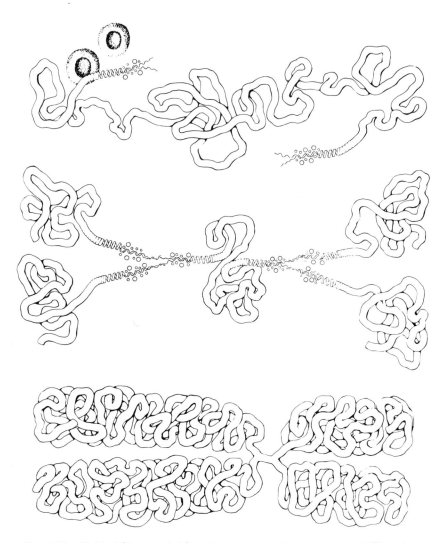

Fig. 5-23.   Folded-fiber model for chromosome ultrastructure in different stages of condensation during mitosis. (Courtesy of E. J. DuPraw, *Nature* 206:338, 1965.)

beginning at the ends and moving to the center. This phenomenon is not generally the case, however.

Watson and Crick considered that the uncoiling was a problem. Our longest human chromosome has a double helix 73,000 μ long. Each turn in Watson-Crick's model is 34 nm so that to uncoil, this chromosome would require 20 million turns!

Theoretical calculations by Levinthal and Crane (1956) estimated that about 1.2×10^{-22} kcal are required to unwind one turn of the DNA molecule. This is quite small as compared to the energy required for the synthesis of DNA. Each turn has ten pairs of bases, requiring 3.3×10^{-19} kcal for the synthesis of one turn from the nucleotides.

Still this does not tell us if the unwinding could go fast enough. Other theoretical calculations by Longuet-Higging and Zimm (1960) suggested that it takes about 1.4 seconds to unwind a piece of double-stranded DNA 5 μ long, containing 15,000 nucleotide pairs. The time grows exponentially with the size.

The rate of biosynthesis has been estimated with radioautography by rate of incorporation of nucleotides to be about 0.5 to 2 μ/min. or 300 to 1,200 nucleotides per minute.

At a rate of 2 μ/min., a human cell with 1,740,000 μ of DNA would require 870,000 minutes to replicate. As in reality it takes less than ten hours, we must assume at least 2,000 points at which replications begin simultaneously.

DNA Polymerase

How would you search for enzyme(s) responsible for DNA replication? What assay would you perform, and what properties would you expect for the system?

This challenge was accepted by Kornberg, who, in 1966, isolated from *E. coli* a new enzyme, DNA polymerase, which catalyzes the reaction:

$$d\text{-ATP} + d\text{-TTP} + d\text{-GTP} + d\text{-CTP} \longrightarrow DNA + n \text{ pyrophosphate}$$

The enzyme is very large, having a molecular weight of 109,000, and consists of a single chain of about 1,000 amino acids. The reaction requires the simultaneous presence of all four nucleotides and of denatured (single-stranded) DNA with at least one free 3'-OH group. One role for the denatured DNA is to act as a *primer*. The new chain is built by consecutive addition of nucleotides to the 3'-OH end (Fig. 5-24). Small deoxynucleotide chains may be added in vitro to perform this primer function. In the presence of a long DNA chain, the newly formed DNA has the same base composition as this added DNA (Fig. 5-25). This indicates that the added DNA has acted as a *template*. Each one of the two complementary DNA chains provides information for the successive addition of nucleotides to the primer, which grows as a complementary DNA chain.

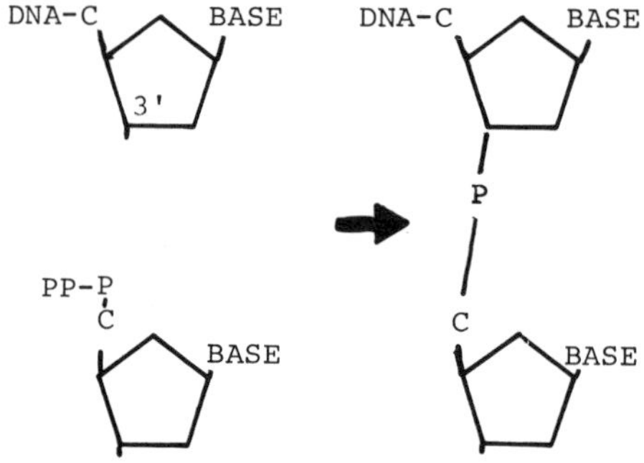

Fig. 5-24. DNA biosynthesis by consecutive addition of nucleotides.

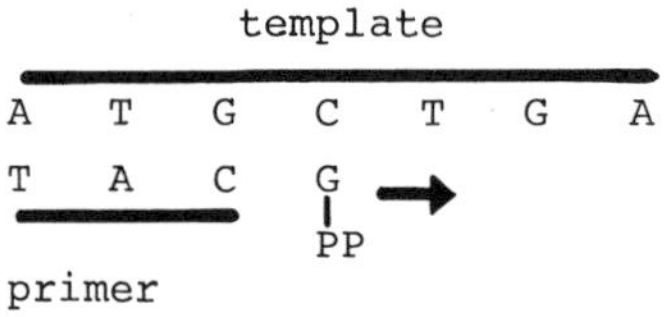

Fig. 5-25. Role of the primer and template in DNA replication.

Finding the same gross base composition is not enough evidence to prove that DNA has replicated. No sequence analysis was available for DNA when Kornberg was carrying out his experiments, so he resorted to a very ingenious method called the *nearest-neighbor analysis.* DNA is synthesized using one of the four nucleotides labeled with ^{32}P in the alpha-phosphate of the nucleotide. The DNA is then hydrolyzed by a bacterial DNAse into 3'-nucleotides (Fig. 5-26). The 5'-^{32}P-labeled phosphate is transferred to the 3' position of its nearest neighbor. Using alpha-^{32}P-labeled ATP, it is possible to measure the relative proportion of ApA, GpA, TpA, and CpA sequences. This is repeated with the other nucleotides, providing relative proportions for 16 dinucleotides. Different values were obtained using different DNAs as templates. Kornberg also isolated the newly formed DNA and reutilized it as a template to obtain a "second-generation" DNA. The nearest-neighbor analysis showed that both the template and the product had the same composition.

If Watson and Crick's model was correct, the newly formed DNA chain should be complementary by the nearest-neighbor analysis. If the newly formed chain was of the same polarity, we should expect GpT =CpA. Analysis revealed equivalent amounts of GpT and ApC (see Figure 5-27), showing that the chain was indeed complementary.

Careful analysis of the polymerase product showed that the main product is a highly ramified DNA with several "hairpin" folds that does not denature when heated. It was shown that polymerase can repair partially hydrolyzed strands or can use a single strand as a primer template (Fig. 5-28).

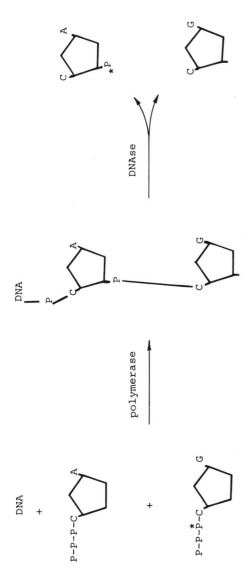

Fig. 5-26. Nearest-neighbor analysis. P* = ³²P-labeled phosphate group.

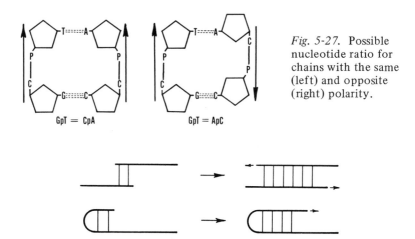

Fig. 5-27. Possible nucleotide ratio for chains with the same (left) and opposite (right) polarity.

Fig. 5-28. Products of synthesis by DNA polymerase in vitro.

DNA polymerase acts also as a DNAse. It was shown that, using a double-stranded DNA with a few *nicks* (points of hydrolysis with free 3'-hydroxyl groups), it can repair the double helix by successively removing nucleotides and replacing them as the DNA chain grows (Fig. 5-29).

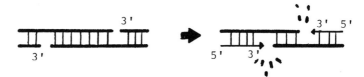

Fig. 5-29. Repair of "nicked" DNA by polymerase.

Autoradiographic studies in *E. coli* showed that DNA replication started at one point and moved steadily in one direction with the simultaneous formation of two chains. DNA polymerase acted only in the 5'–3' direction, and as the chains were of opposed polarity, it could not replicate both chains. A great effort was made to find another DNA polymerase that could act in the reverse direction, so that by combining the action of both enzymes, the DNA could replicate starting at one point. Neither such another enzyme nor 3'-triphosphates nor diphosphates were found to exist in the cell.

Kornberg proposed that DNA replication was a concerted action of three different enzymes. According to his idea, a nick is initially produced by an endonuclease. DNA polymerase then makes first one strand, then a second, producing a fork (Fig. 5-30). The fork is then cleaved by the endonuclease, providing a new point for replication. This results in a number of small chains which must be linked together.

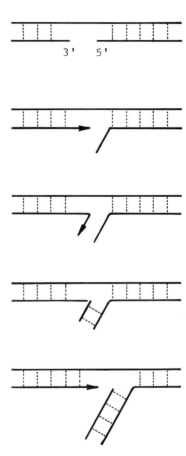

Fig. 5-30. DNA replication by synthesis of two strands by DNA polymerase.

Using radioactive isotopes, it was possible to demonstrate that a number of small strands $(1-2\ \mu)$ of DNA are formed as predicted by this model. Moreover, enzymes that can link these small strands were discovered. They are called *selases* or *ligases*. They catalyze the reaction

nicked DNA + ATP ⟶ DNA + AMP + PP

nicked DNA + NAD ⟶ DNA + AMP + NMN

There are some mutants of *E. coli* that can be maintained in culture but are very sensitive to ultraviolet radiations. It was found that those mutants do not contain DNA polymerase, which suggests that this enzyme is not required for DNA replication.

Ultraviolet radiation damages DNA by producing chemical changes in thymidine, with the formation of a covalent bond between two close thymidines. This bond, linking across the two DNA chains, interferes with unwinding and replication. There is an ultraviolet repair enzyme that removes the thymidine dimers, leaving behind a broken DNA. DNA polymerase is required to repair this DNA, which explains why some DNA polymerase–lacking mutants are very sensitive to ultraviolet radiations. It was found recently that xeroderma pigmentosum, a rare hereditary disease that results in hypersensitivity of the skin to sunlight, is due to the lack of the DNA repair enzyme system.

Another DNA polymerase, membrane-bound, was found in mutants, and it seems possible that this is the real enzyme involved in chromosomal replication. There are strong indications that bacterial chromosomes are attached to the bacterial membrane, and in eukaryotic cells (cells with a nucleus), chromosomes are attached to the nuclear membrane. It is possible that replication begins at these points.

Recently it was shown that RNA can act as a primer for DNA replication. It is possible that this is accomplished through special small RNA strands produced at the replication points. Another group of proteins presently under active investigation seem to be capable of unwinding supercoils of DNA. It is not impossible that there is a quite different enzyme system for replication, and that the function of polymerase is restricted to repair. This may be true even though it is possible, with DNA polymerase, endonuclease, and a ligase, to replicate in a test tube a DNA virus which is infective and is capable of initiating and continuing reproduction of new virions in cells.

TRANSCRIBING THE MESSAGE

The relationship between genetic information and proteins emerged slowly. In the beginning of this century, a lecture was presented at the Royal College of Physicians in England which was a landmark in medical and biological sciences. Garrod discussed "inborn errors of metabolism," showing that several human diseases, rare and hereditary, were associated with metabolic defects. These included alkaptonuria, which is characterized by excretion of a compound in urine which becomes dark on contact with air, and albinism, which is caused by incapability to produce melanin. It was only in 1941 that the genetic control of enzymes became realizable in the laboratory, when Beadle and Tatum began study of the mutants of the mold Neurospora. Their "one gene—one enzyme" theory was recognized by the presentation of a Nobel prize.

From medical science came another breakthrough when, in 1949, Pauling proposed that sickle cell anemia was a molecular disease. When Ingram located the single amino acid error, stronger evidence was provided for the belief that genetic information must code for the primary structure of proteins in general.

Red cells continue to make hemoglobin after the nucleus disappears. In 1951 Brachet and Chantrene used the sea alga, *Acetabularia,* to investigate the role of the nucleus. Upon cutting out the base, they found that the rest of the cell continued to live for some time. It did not make a significant amount of nucleic acids, but it continued to incorporate amino acids into proteins.

Goldstein and Plaut, in 1955, did some fascinating experiments using amoebas and microsurgery. They raised some amoebas on a diet of ^{32}P-labeled microorganisms in order to label the amoebas' nuclei. When these nuclei were transplanted to other amoebas, autoradiography revealed that ^{32}P label moved into the cytoplasm. The labeled compound could be removed by treating the preparations with RNAse before the autoradiography, showing that the compound was RNA. Further work by Goldstein demonstrated that proteins can migrate from the cytoplasm into the nucleus but do not migrate in the reverse direction.

What can be concluded from these experiments? Where are proteins synthesized? How is information provided for this synthesis?

Cytochemical studies have shown that rapidly growing cells, or cells with active protein synthesis, make large amounts of RNA with a rapid turnover. Crick proposed in 1957 that genetic information is carried out to the cytoplasm by a nuclear-made RNA which today we call *mRNA,* or *messenger RNA.*

Back in 1955, Grunberg-Manago and Ochoa discovered what appeared to be the enzyme that made RNA. It synthesizes RNA from a mixture of ribonucleotide diphosphates: adenosine diphosphate (ADP), guanosine diphosphate (GDP), cytidine diphosphate (CDP), and uridyl diphosphate (UDP). This came like a bomb — nucleic acid could be made in the test tube with an isolated purified enzyme! It turned out that this enzyme is probably involved in the hydrolysis of RNA, not in its synthesis. It can catalyze in the reverse direction to make a random polymer according to the supply of diphosphonucleotides, without any order or specificity. Still, this discovery proved to be a fundamental step in helping to unveil the mystery of the genetic code. It showed that the traditional approach of searching for an enzyme, isolating it in pure form, and studying its properties was possible in nucleic acid synthesis systems. Ochoa's enzyme was an invaluable tool in the production of artificial RNA of known base composition for molecular biology.

Five years later, several laboratories showed that another enzyme existed in plants, bacteria, and animal cells for RNA synthesis.

What are the properties you would investigate to convince yourself that this enzyme transfers information from DNA to RNA? Study the results obtained by Hurwitz and decide if this RNA polymerase is the enzyme actually involved in the synthesis of mRNA.

THE ENZYMATIC INCORPORATION OF RIBONUCLEOTIDES INTO RNA AND THE ROLE OF DNA (Tables)

Jerard Hurwitz, J. J. Furth, Monika Anders, P. J. Ortiz, and J. T. August

Table 1. Requirement for Incorporation Substrate GR-P^{32}-P-P

Addition	mumole incorporated/20′
1. Complete	0.57
2. Omit 1 or 3 Nucleoside Triphosphates	<0.01
3. Omit DNA	<0.01
4. RNA in place of DNA	<0.01
5. Omit Mg^{++} and Mn^{++}	<0.01
6. Preincubation with DNase for 30′	<0.01

The reaction mixture (0.5 ml) contained P^{32}-GTP (1×10^6 cpm/μM) 20 mumoles; ATP, UTP and GTP, 50 mumoles of each; thymus DNA, 1 optical density unit at 260 mu; Tris buffer, pH 7.5, 20 μmoles; MgCl$_2$, 4 μmoles; MnCl$_2$, 2 μmoles; mercaptoethylamine, 1 μmole; Ammonium Sulfate II, 4 μg. Where indicated, 2 to 5 optical density units (at 260 mu) of TMV-RNA or *E. coli* ribosomal RNA or yeast or *E. coli* soluble RNA was used in place of DNA.

Table 3. Hydrolysis of Product by RNAse and Alkali

	Acid-Insoluble, cpm
1. No treatment—20′ at 38°	1550
2. DNase (1 μg)— ″ ″ ″	1450
3. RNase (1 μg)— ″ ″ ″	<20
4. NaOH (1 M for 12 hrs)	<20

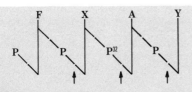

Fig. 2. Alkaline transfer reaction with RNA.

Table 4. Distribution of P^{32} After Alkaline Degradation (Thymus DNA as Primer)

Labeled Nucleotide	% Distribution of P^{32} After Alkaline Degradation			
	Ap	Cp	Gp	Up
AP*-PP	38	18	27	17
UP*-PP	24	24	17	35
CP*-P-P	22	21	21	36
GP*-P-P	21	18	21	40

The conditions used were as described in Table 1. The products were isolated by acid precipitation and subjected to alkaline degradation. The 2′(3′) mononucleotides were then separated by electrophoresis.

Table 5. Stoichiometry of Incorporation of the Four Nucleotides

	Incorporated mumoles
1. C^{14}-ATP + UTP + GTP + CTP	21.4
2. ATP + C^{14}-UTP + GTP + CTP	19.6
3. ATP + UTP + P^{32}-GTP + CTP	16.8
4. ATP + UTP + GTP + P^{32}-CTP	17.0
Sum	74.8
Total increase in acid-insoluble orcinol material	81.5

The incubation mixture and assay were as described in Table 1 except that the additions were increased 10-fold.

Table 6. Requirements for Release of Radioactivity from UR-P P* P

	mumoles
1. Complete system	1.18
2. Omit DNA	0.14
3. Omit either ATP or GTP or CTP	0.24
4. Omit Mn^{++}	1.31

All conditions were as described in Table 1 except that β-P^{32} UTP was used. The reaction was terminated with acid, and the nucleic acid removed by centrifugation. The supernatant solutions were then treated with 0.1 ml of a 30% suspension of charcoal which was washed 3 times by centrifugation and resuspension. The charcoal was suspended in 1.0 ml of an ethanolic NH_3-H_2O solution, plated, and its radioactivity measured.

Table 7. Influence of Different DNA Preparations on Incorporation of Nucleotides

DNA Added	Nucleotide Incorporation in mμmoles						
	$\dfrac{A+T}{C+G}$ reported	AMP	UMP	GMP	CMP	$\dfrac{A+U}{C+G}$ observed	$\dfrac{A+G}{U+C}$
T2-DNA	1.86	0.54	0.59	0.31	0.30	1.85	0.96
Thymus-DNA	1.35	3.10	3.30	2.0	2.2	1.52	0.93
E. coli DNA	1.0	2.70	2.74	2.90	2.94	0.93	0.98
Micrococcus DNA	0.40	0.55	0.52	1.10	1.12	0.48	1.01

The complete system contained: ATP, GTP, CTP, and UTP (50 mumoles each), $MgCl_2$ (4 μmoles), $MnCl_2$ (2 μmoles), mercaptoethylamine (1 μmole), Tris buffer (25 μmoles, pH 7.5), 12 to 24 μg of protein and DNA. The DNA additions were as follows: T2—0.56 optical density units at 260 mu and Mn^{++} was omitted; thymus, 1 optical density unit; *E. coli,* 1 optical density unit; *Micrococcus* DNA, 1 optical density unit.

The observation that virus ϕX-174 DNA primed the incorporation of ribonucleotides was of particular interest because this DNA, in contrast to the DNA preparations previously described, is single-stranded.

Table 8. Base Composition of RNA Using ϕX-174 DNA as Primer

Nucleotide Incorporated	Mumoles per 20 min.	Base Ratio	
		Observed	Theoretical*
AMP	1.02	1.25	1.33
UMP	0.82	1	1
CMP	0.75	0.91	0.98
GMP	0.66	0.80	0.75

ϕX-174 DNA = 0.1 optical density unit at 250 mu; all other additions were as described in Table 1.
*Theoretical ratio is based on Sinsheimer's reported ratio of A = 1, T = 1.33, G = 0.98, C = 0.75.

Table 9. Requirements for AMP Incorporation with Poly T and Thymus DNA as Primers

Additions	Thymus DNA	Poly T
	mμmoles incorporated	
1. Complete System	1.47	4.25
2. Omit GTP, UTP and CTP	0.15	6.80
3. 1 +RNAse (5 μg)	0.22	–
4. 2 +RNAse (5 μg)	–	7.0
5. 1 +DNAse (5 μg)	0.18	–
6. 2 +DNAse (5 μg)	–	2.84

The following additions were made: C^{14}-ATP (50 mumoles), GTP, UTP and CTP (80 mumoles each), Poly T (0.5 optical density units at 250 mu), $MgCl_2$ (4 μmoles), $MnCl_2$ (2 μmoles), mercaptoethylamine (1 μmole), Tris buffer (25 μmoles, pH 7.5) and 12 μg of a 100-fold purified enzyme preparation obtained from *E. coli* W.

RNase and DNase were added before the *E. coli* enzyme. If DNA were pretreated with DNase, no detectable acid-insoluble radioactivity was found.

Table 10. Specificity of Poly T and Thymus DNA in Governing Nucleotide Incorporation

	Labeled Precursor Incorporated			
	C^{14}-AMP	P^{32}-GMP	P^{32}-UMP	P^{32}-CMP
	mμmoles incorporated			
Thymus DNA + Complete System	1.95	1.40	1.06	1.20
Poly T + Complete System	4.4	0.05	0.11	<0.02
Poly T + labeled nucleotide only	6.15	0.09	<0.02	<0.02

The complete system contained 40 mumoles each of all 4 nucleoside triphosphates with one labeled as indicated. The specific activities (cpm per μmole) of the labeled nucleotides were: C^{14}-ATP, 1.95×10^6; GTP^{32}, 1.78×10^6; UTP^{32}, 0.64×10^6; CTP, 1.66×10^6. All other additions were as described in Table 9.

Table 11. Specificity of the D-AT Copolymer as Primer

Labeled precursor as substrate	mμmoles incorporated
C^{14}-ATP	0.97
C^{14}-UTP	1.10
P^{32}-GTP	<.03
P^{32}-CTP	<.03
C^{14}-UTP (omit CTP and GTP)	1.06

The additions were as follows: $MgCl_2$ (4 μmoles), $MnCl_2$ (2 μmoles), mercaptoethanol (1 μmole), Tris buffer pH 7.5 (25 μmoles), d-AT copolymer (0.22 optical density units at 262 mu), 12 μg of a 100-fold purified enzyme preparation and all 4 ribonucleoside triphosphates. One of the nucleoside triphosphates was labeled with either C^{14} or P^{32} in the a-phosphate group. The amounts and specific activities of the labeled nucleotides were: C^{14}-ATP, 5- mumoles (1950 cpm/mumole), C^{14}-UTP, 21 mumoles (637 cpm/mumole), P^{32}-GTP, 41 mumoles (780 cpm/mumole) and P^{32}-CTP, 35 mumoles (738 cpm/mumole). 80 mumoles of the three other nucleoside triphosphates were added in each experiment except where otherwise indicated.

Table 12. Requirements for AMP and UMP Incorporation with the D-AT Copolymer as Primer

Additions	mμmoles incorporated
C^{14}-ATP + UTP	1.0
C^{14}-ATP, omit UTP	0.17
C^{14}-UTP + ATP	1.03
C^{14}-UTP, omit ATP	<0.04

The additions were as in Table 11 except that the nucleoside triphosphates were added as indicated, CTP and GTP were omitted, and 0.11 optical density units of d-AT copolymer were added. The reaction was terminated after 20 minutes.

Table 13. Distribution of P^{32} Following Alkaline Degradation of the Product Prepared Using the d-AT Copolymer as Primer

Substrates	mμmoles Incorporated	Distribution of Radioactivity after alkaline hydrolysis (%)			
		AMP	CMP	GMP	UMP
$AP^{32}PP$ + UTP	16.3	6	<0.5	<0.5	94
ATP + $UP^{32}PP$	19.5	100	<0.5	<0.5	<0.5

The reaction vessels contained (in 5.0 ml) either 400 mumoles of AP^{32}-PP (765 cpm/mumole) plus 800 mumoles of UTP or 472 mumoles of UP^{32}-PP (242 cpm/mumole) plus 800 mumoles of ATP. Both contained d-AT copolymer (0.44 optical density units), MgCl$_2$ (40 μmoles), MnCl$_2$ (20 μmoles), Tris buffer, pH 7.5 (250 μmoles), mercaptoethanol (10 μmoles) and 120 μg of enzyme protein. After 30 minutes at 38°, the reaction was stopped with perchloric acid and 1.2 mg of bovine serum albumin were added. The acid-insoluble material was washed with 1%

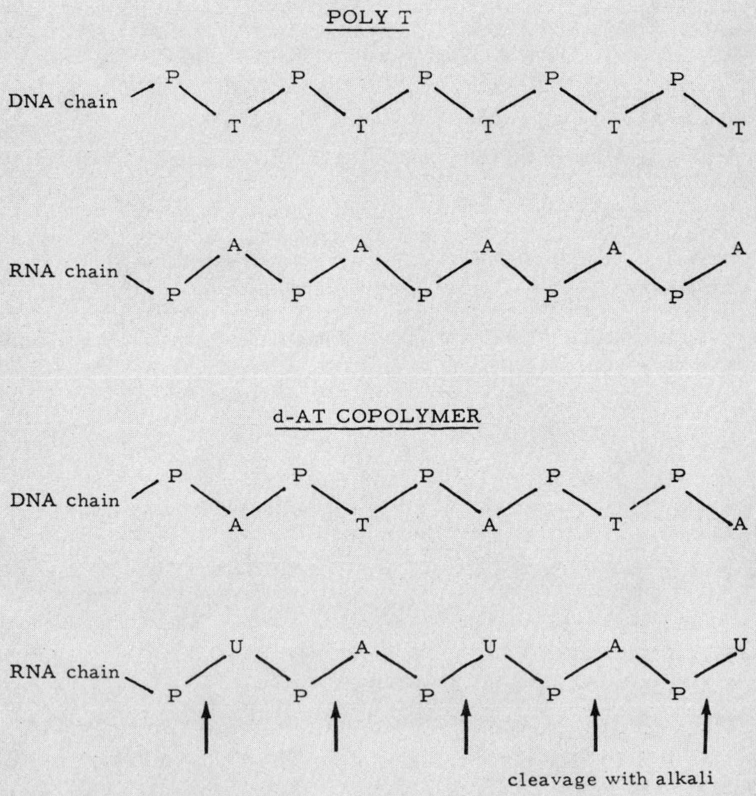

Fig. 3. Results with Poly T and d-AT Copolymer as Primers.

perchloric acid, dissolved in 1.5 ml of 1N NaOH and incubated for 16 hours at 38°
The hydrolysates were then adsorbed to Norit, washed with water, and the nucleotides eluted with ethanolic-NH_3. The nucleotides plus carrier amounts of each of
the $2'(3')$ mononucleotides were then fractionated by paper electrophoresis, located
by ultraviolet light examination, eluted with water and their radioactivity determined.

Approximately 75% of the radioactivity in the alkaline hydrolysate was eluted
from Norit. The elution of the material after paper electrophoresis was quantitative. The amounts of the alkaline hydrolysate used for electrophoresis were 2.53
and 3.94 mumoles for the experiments with AP^{32}-PP and UP^{32}-PP, respectively.

Table 15. Product Sensitivity to DNase and RNase

	Time of Incubation	
Treatment of Product	15'	30'
	Acid-insoluble Radioactivity, cpm	
A. Phenol Isolated Product		
1. No addition	475	450
2. DNAse (5 µg)	450	435
3. RNAse (5 µg)	200	175
4. RNAse + DNase	200	175
B. Phenol Product Heated at 100° or Acid-treated		
1. No addition	450	420
2. DNase	420	400
3. RNase	<50	<50

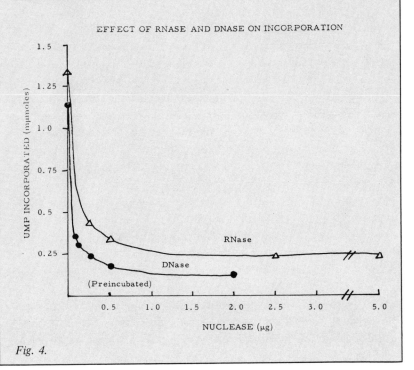

EFFECT OF RNASE AND DNASE ON INCORPORATION

Fig. 4.

(From Cold Springs Harbor Symposia on
Quantitative Biology, *Vol. 26, 1961.)*

HYBRIDIZATION

In 1960, Hall and Spiegelman discovered a new technique that would revolutionize molecular biology. They infected bacteria with a virus, providing ^{3}H-thymidine in the medium. From the bacteria they isolated the virus DNA with the ^{3}H label. In a parallel experiment, they provided a medium containing ^{32}P-phosphate and isolated the newly formed ^{32}P-RNA. They showed that, upon mixing RNA with the denatured DNA, a hybrid DNA-RNA molecule appeared that could be isolated by using density gradient centrifugation. DNA from other species did not hybridize to the same order of magnitude. Using a purified RNA, they showed that the hybridization increased with the concentration of RNA until it reached a saturation point. Adding different RNA from the same species resulted in further hybridization, proving that each RNA hybridizes with its corresponding DNA.

The hybridization method has been considerably simplified and is now easy to run. Each week, there are dozens of papers published reporting new data using this technique. DNA is trapped in a cellulose filter and radioactive RNA is filtered through it. All the RNA that hybridizes is retained on the filter and can thus be counted.

Using hybridization techniques, it was shown that although RNA polymerase transcribes both DNA strands in vitro, in vivo it transcribes only one of the strands along any particular segment of DNA.

RNA polymerase starts synthesis at the 5′ end. It is made of several different polypeptide chains, one being easily dissociated — the sigma factor. In the absence of the sigma factor, the enzyme is capable of synthesis but produces a number of incomplete transcriptions of different lengths; transcription is random. The sigma factor seems to be essential for the enzyme to recognize the beginning of the message. It has been postulated that there are more factors of this type, which make possible the recognition of different DNAs as well as recognition of cellular DNA as opposed to that brought in by viruses which are parasites on the host.

Actinomycin D (Fig. 5-31) is a very toxic antibiotic. It can bind to DNA (by hydrogen bonding with guanine), completely blocking transcription by RNA polymerase. Another antibiotic, rifamycin, also blocks RNA polymerase. These two inhibitors are very important tools in the study of the role of transcription in biological processes: they enable investigators to see if a biological process requires the synthesis of a new messenger RNA.

Rich's investigations (1956–1960) showed that the double helix forms spontaneously on mixing of polydeoxyribonucleotides, or of polydeoxyribonucleotides and polyribonucleotides with complementary bases, as predicted by

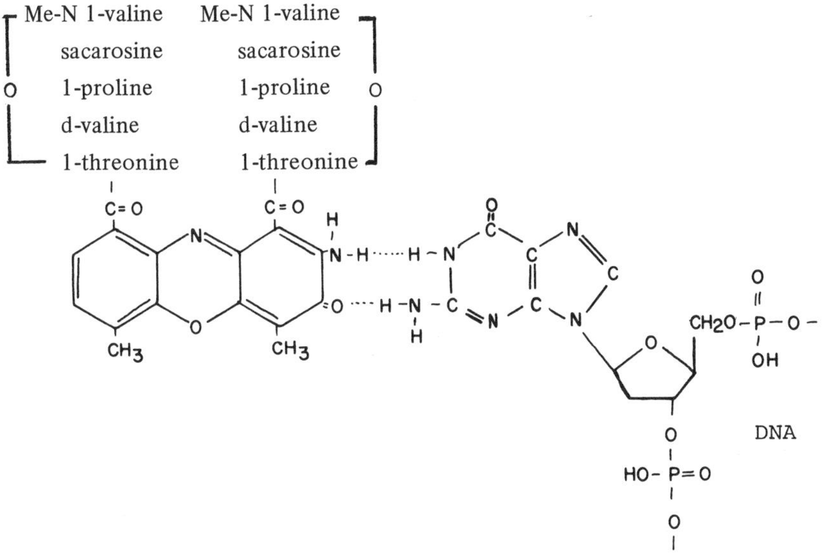
Me-N 1-valine
sacarosine
1-proline
d-valine
1-threonine
Me-N 1-valine
sacarosine
1-proline
d-valine
1-threonine
O
O
C=O
C=O
N
O
CH3
CH3
N-H
H-N
O
H-N-C
N
C
C
C
N
C
N
O
CH2O-P-O-
OH
O
HO-P=O
O
DNA

Fig. 5-31. Actinomycin D.

Watson and Crick. In 1960, Dotty and Marmour found that natural, denatured DNA can renature spontaneously, if left to cool very slowly. This provided a new means of comparing DNAs from different origins. By mixing denatured DNA from two species and comparing the percentages of pairing, we gain some idea of the common nucleotide sequences. As expected, the closer the species are morphologically, the greater the number of common sequences (Fig. 5-32).

THE ROLE OF SOLUBLE RNA

Early cytologists noticed that the cytoplasm of a cell that synthesizes large amounts of protein (e.g., glandular cells that make large quantities of particular enzymes and hormones or the bone marrow cells that make hemoglobin) is stained by *basophilic* stains. These reagents combine with acidic compounds, and cytochemistry showed that they were RNA. With the development of electron microscopy, the apparently structureless cytoplasm was shown to contain a multifolded membrane with a number of specialized organelles (Fig. 5-33). This multifolded membrane was named the *endoplasmic reticulum,* and was shown to be lined by small bodies called *ribosomes.*

The broken cells obtained by homogenizing the tissue in isotonic sucrose are capable of continuing protein synthesis, as measured by incorporation of

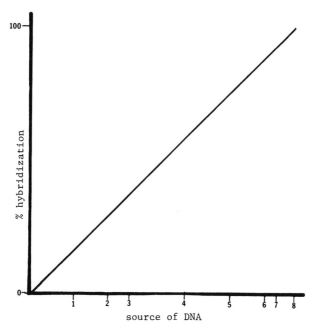

Fig. 5-32. Homology of DNA in different mammals: (1) hedgehog, (2) tree shrew, (3) lemur, (4) tarsir, (5) capuchin monkey, (6) gibbon, (7) chimpanzee, (8) man.

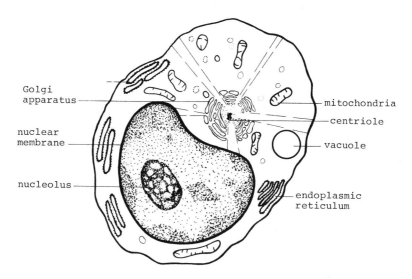

Fig. 5-33. Schematic diagram of an animal cell.

radioactive amino acids into proteins. Using centrifugation, it is possible to isolate from the homogenate the three insoluble fractions — nucleus, mitochondria, and microsomes — leaving behind the cell supernatant with the soluble materials. Microsomal fractions are made from the minced parts of the endoplasmic reticulum. In 1952, Siekevitz showed that amino acid incorporation requires the microsomal fraction, the cell supernatant, and mitochondria or some source of ATP. Treating the microsomal fraction with deoxycholate causes the membrane to dissolve, freeing ribosomes which can still incorporate amino acids.

In 1958, Hoagland and Zamecnik resolved this system further. They showed that GTP was required along with ATP and that the cell supernatant supplied an enzyme (called *enzyme 5.4*) and soluble RNA. The enzyme was shown to activate amino acids by combining them with RNA:

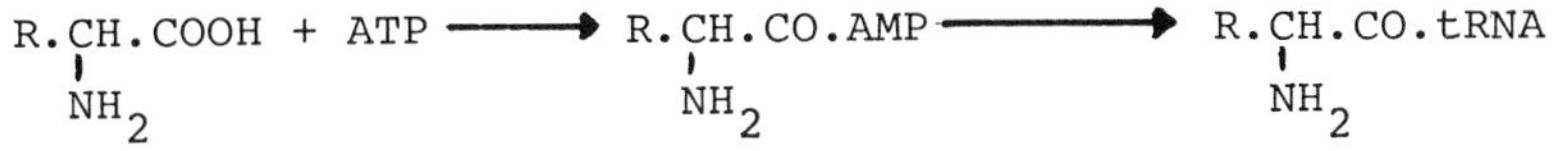

$$R.\underset{\underset{NH_2}{|}}{CH}.COOH + ATP \longrightarrow R.\underset{\underset{NH_2}{|}}{CH}.CO.AMP \longrightarrow R.\underset{\underset{NH_2}{|}}{CH}.CO.tRNA$$

Fig. 5-34. Amino acid activation for protein synthesis.

The enzyme 5.4 and the soluble RNA were resolved into a large number of enzymes and RNAs that could specifically activate a single amino acid. In most organisms, more than one RNA was found for a single amino acid.

The soluble RNAs were shown to be small, with about 70 to 80 nucleotides. Some of these nucleotides are modified by methylation or by attached SH groups. About 25 such modified nucleotides have been identified. Their identification gave a polynucleotide sequence with many markers which allowed Holey, in 1966, to use different methods to break up the chain into small sequences and identify them. This work, similar to the initial work of Sanger in sequencing the amino acids of insulin, made possible the revelation of the total primary structure of a nucleic acid for the first time (Fig. 5-35).

Today the primary sequence of nucleotides of about fifteen soluble RNAs has been determined. Each one has been found to have a phosphate at the $5'$ end, generally with guanine, and OH–ACC at the $3'$ end. G_2^2m and a sequence TΨC are also common to all those molecules (Fig. 5-36). Several secondary structures have been proposed, built on pairing of complementary bases. The most popular is the "cloverleaf," with three large loops and a fourth of variable length containing 4 to 21 nucleotides. Recently, Rich et al. have completed x-ray diffraction studies on one of these RNAs, showing a complex tridimensional tertiary structure.

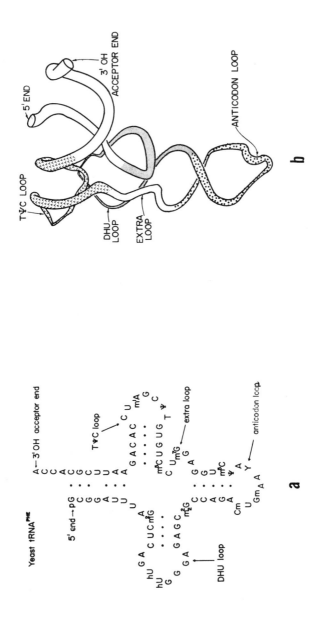

Fig. 5-35. (a) Sequence of nucleotides and cloverleaf diagram of yeast tRNA for phenylalanine. (b) Structure of yeast tRNA for phenylalanine. (Courtesy of S. H. Kim et al., *Science* 179:285, 1973.)

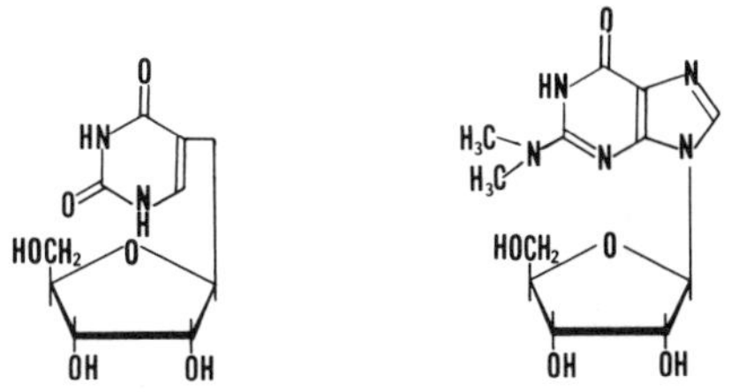

Fig. 5-36. Nitrogen bases common to tRNA.

4 pseudouridine

Ψ

dimethyl guanosine

G_2^2m

In the synthesis of proteins, amino acids must be ordered and combined in the proper sequence if they are to produce a functional protein. Crick proposed that to recognize the information coded by the messenger RNA, an RNA adaptor must exist which can recognize the information and can order the amino acids for peptide linking.

The soluble RNAs fit this prediction very well. It was shown that different RNAs combined specifically with amino acids and that the RNA-bound amino acids were transferred to the newly formed proteins on the ribosome. Thus, the soluble RNAs became known as *transfer RNA,* or *tRNA.* Still, a demonstration was needed to show that ordering is due to recognition of the coded messenger RNA *(mRNA)* by the tRNA. In 1962, Chappeville, Lipman, and their co-workers performed a conclusive experiment. They charged the cysteine-tRNA with ^{14}C-cysteine. By chemical treatment, the bound cysteine was transformed into alanine by removing the SH group. When this alanyl-tRNA was used for protein synthesis, it was shown that the alanine replaced cysteine, proving that the code resided in the tRNA and that the *codon* in the mRNA should have a corresponding *anticodon* in the tRNA. This anticodon recognizes the codon by complementary pairing of the bases.

RIBOSOMES AND PROTEIN SYNTHESIS

In 1961, Dintzis treated rabbits with phenylhydrazine, inducing the release into the bloodstream of reticulocytes actively synthesizing hemoglobin. From these reticulocytes he prepared ribosomes, which he incubated for different lengths of time with ^{3}H-leucine. The soluble hemoglobin released was dissociated into alpha and beta chains, which were each hydrolyzed into peptides. The relative amount of tritium in each chain was measured (Fig. 5-38).

Dintzis proposed a model for protein synthesis as shown in Figure 5-37.

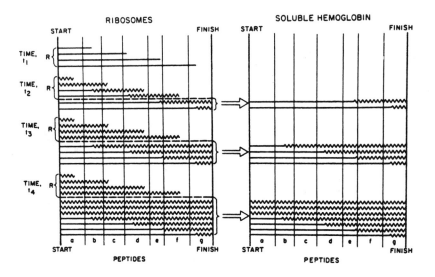

Fig. 5-37. Model of sequential chain growth. The straight lines represent unlabeled polypeptide chain. The zigzag lines represent radioactively labeled polypeptide chain formed after the addition of radioactive amino acid at time t_1. The groups of peptides labeled R are those unfinished bits attached to the ribosomes at each time; the rest, having reached the finish line, are assumed to be present in the soluble hemoglobin. In the ribosome at time t_2, the top two completely zigzag lines represent peptide chains formed completely from amino acids during the time interval between t_1 and t_2. The middle two lines represent chains which have grown during the time interval but have not reached the finish line and are therefore still attached to the ribosomes. The bottom two chains represent those which have crossed the finish line, left the ribosomes, and are to be found mixed with other molecules of soluble hemoglobin. (Courtesy H. M. Dintzis, *Proc. Nat. Acad. Sci.* 47:247, 1961.)

This and other studies demonstrated that proteins are synthesized by step-wise elongation from the amino end. Dintzis's data suggest a rate of approximately two amino acids per second.

This process requires a subcellular structure — the ribosome. Animal ribosomes are spherical in shape, with a diameter of about 22 nm and a molecular weight of 4 million. Their sedimentation constant in the ultracentrifuge is 80S. (This number is more commonly used than the molecular weight.)

At low magnesium concentrations, the 80S ribosomes dissociate into two different subunits: a 60S and a 40S particle. The 60S particle contains about 40 different proteins and a 28S RNA and a 18S RNA with molecular weights of about 2×10^6 and 3×10^4, respectively. The 40S particle contains about 20 different proteins and an 18S RNA with a molecular weight of 7×10^5.

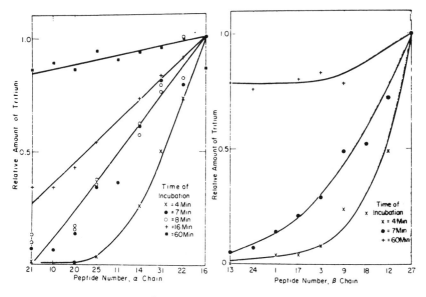

Fig. 5-38. Distribution of ^{3}H-leucine among tryptic peptides of soluble rabbit hemoglobin after various times of incubation at 15° C. (Courtesy of H. M. Dintzis, *Proc. Nat. Acad. Sci.* 47:247, 1961.)

Bacterial ribosomes are smaller (70S, 18nm) with proportionally smaller particles (50S and 30S) and RNA (23S and 16S).

In 1963, Rich incubated reticulocytes with ^{14}C amino acids. He broke the reticulocytes gently in a hypotonic medium and layered them in a sucrose gradient that was submitted to ultracentrifugation. He punctured the bottom of the tube and collected fractions from the more dense to the less dense parts of the suspension. Each fraction was analyzed for its protein content, its absorption at 250 nm, and the amount of ^{14}C incorporation by radioactive counting.

Examine the two figures (5-39, 5-40) from the original paper. What would you conclude?

It is seen in Figure 5-39 that gently treated cell lysates have, besides the ribosomes (around tube 30, corresponding to about 78S), a much larger particle (tube 17 with 170S). Less gently treated lysates have several particles of intermediate size. Incorporation of amino acids does not occur in the ribosomes but rather in the larger particles. Figure 5-40 shows that the large particles can be broken down into ribosomes, with bound ^{14}C-incorporated

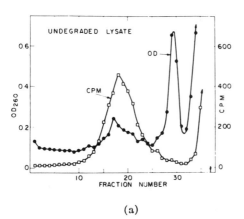

(a)

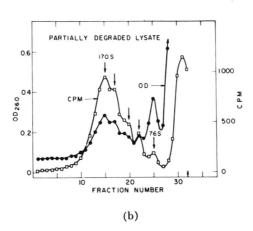

(b)

Fig. 5-39. Sucrose gradients of lysed reticulocytes after a short incubation with ^{14}C amino acids. 1 ml. of lysate was layered on 25 ml of a 15−30% sucrose gradient and then centrifuged (55,000 × g, 2 hours, 25° C). The short vertical arrows in the figure indicate peaks. (a) Undegraded lysate. (b) Partially degraded lysate. CPM = counts per minute; $O.D._{260}$ = optical density at 260 nm. (Courtesy of A. Rich et al., *Proc. Nat. Acad. Sci.* 49:122, 1963.)

amino acids, by RNAse but not by DNAse. Examination of the preparation under the electron microscope showed isolated ribosomes and polysomes made of a cluster of two to six ribosomes. Better preparations with higher resolution show that Rich was correct in assuming that several ribosomes are attached at the same time to a messenger RNA. The mRNA for one hemoglobin chain has been estimated to be a molecule 150 nm long, which can accommodate up to six ribosomes. Electron microscopy shows the ribosomes, ordered with the small subunit to one side, attached to a long, thin strand which is the mRNA.

By using ^{15}N precursors to label the RNA of the ribosomal units and mixing them with unlabeled ribosomes, it was possible to show that they dissociate and reassociate during protein synthesis.

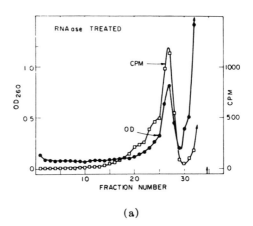

(a)

Fig. 5-40. Sucrose gradients of reticulocyte lysate as in Figure 5-39 but incubated at 4°C for 1 hour with (a) 0.25 µg/ml RNAse: the 170 peak has disappeared and the radioactivity is now in the 76S peak; and (b) 10 µg/ml DNAse: the 76S and 170S peaks are unchanged from Figure 5-39. (Courtesy of A. Rich et al., *Proc. Nat. Acad. Sci.,* 49:122, 1963.)

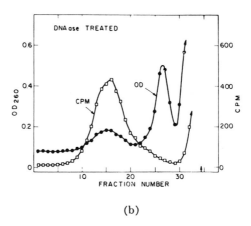

(b)

In *E. coli* it was found that the N-terminal amino acids were not randomly distributed but that methionine was especially frequently found. In 1964, Marcker found that one of the two methionyl-tRNAs was transformed by an enzymatic reaction into formyl-methionyl-tRNA, and that this compound was necessary to initiate protein synthesis.

In the case of hemoglobin, the N-terminal amino group is valine. However, when Dantkis and Wilson (1970) searched for new chains of short length, they found a polypeptide having methionine in the N-terminal end, followed by valine. It seems that, in eukaryotic cells, methionyl-tRNA is necessary to start new protein chains, but in the process of releasing the final protein, methionine can be excised.

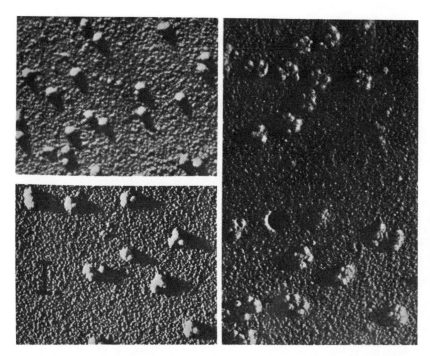

Fig. 5-41. Electron micrographs of reticulocyte ribosomes. The ribosomes were deposited on the grid as a droplet from the sucrose gradient, rinsed with buffer, and air-dried. The platinum shadowing was at a 5:1 angle. The verticle mark indicates 0.1μ. Upper left: Droplet from the 76S peak. Lower left: Droplet from the 134S peak showing triplets of ribosomes. Right: Droplet from the 170S peak showing several ribosome pentamers. (Courtesy of A. Rich et al., *Proc. Nat. Acad. Sci.,* 49:122, 1963.)

By careful washing of the ribosomal preparation, a number of proteins have been identified as participants in the process of protein synthesis. Some are required for the initiation (F_1, F_2, F_3) of new chains in conjunction with methionyl-tRNA, others during the elongation of the chain (T_u, T_s, G) and finally, one factor is involved in the termination as a release factor (R).

A schematic presentation of the process is shown in Figure 5-42. The factors and ribosomes are used to catalyze the process in a cyclic manner as they move along the mRNA reading the information and translating it into a protein structure.

The roles of the ribosomal proteins and RNAs are not clear. The larger subunits provide the peptidyl transferase activity that catalyzes the synthesis

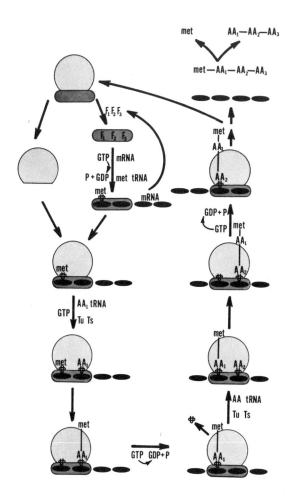

Fig. 5-42. Protein synthesis.

of the peptide bond. Together with factors G and T, the ribosome acts as a mechanical device which moves along the messenger, one step at a time.

It seems probable that, as the protein chain grows, it starts to assume its stable tridimensional shape by the interaction of hydrophobic and hydrogen bonds. It is possible that the methionine end is removed during protein synthesis. In the endoplasmic reticulum there is an enzyme which is responsible for the oxidation of the −SH group with the formation of S-S bonds. This system can, by a mechanism not yet understood, select the proper −SH groups in the case of proteins with more than two, such as insulin and ribonuclease.

Protein synthesis is inhibited by many compounds, including a number of antibiotics (Fig. 5-43). Cycloheximide is active in eukaryotic ribosomes. Chloramphenicol blocks the synthesis by bacteria and in eukaryotic mitochondria. Actually, mitochondria resemble bacteria in several respects; they have their own DNA, small ribosomes similar to those of bacteria, and formyl-methionyl-tRNA as a protein initiator. Another antibiotic, puromycin, resembles aminoacyl-tRNA and reacts to form peptidyl-puromycin, thus stopping further elongation by releasing the peptide.

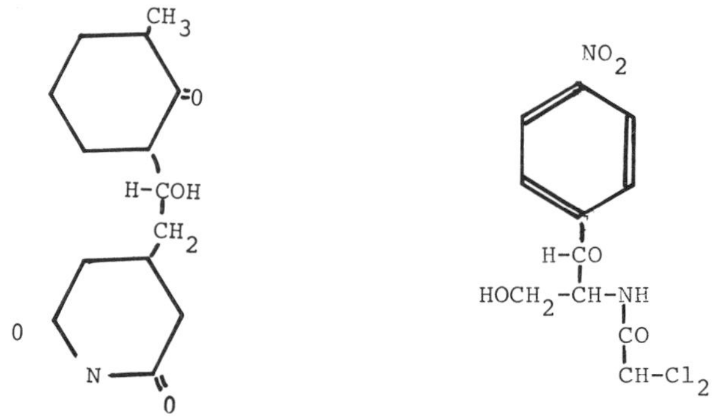

Fig. 5-43. Inhibitors of protein synthesis. Left, cycloheximide; right, chloramphenicol.

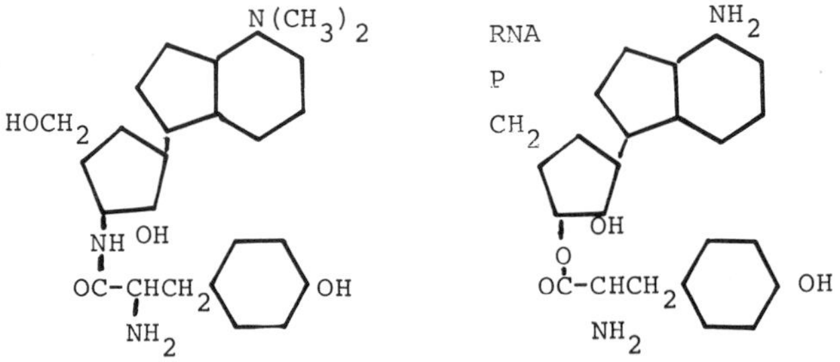

Fig. 5-44. Structural similarity between puromycin (left) and amino acid tRNA (right).

The cycles that associate and release subparticles and factors involved in protein synthesis allow successive reutilization of this complex machinery. The cost of protein synthesis is one molecule of ATP per amino acid bound to tRNA broken into AMP and PP, which in turn is split into inorganic phosphate. At least one molecule of GTP is broken down during the process of elongation per amino acid added. This results in the utilization of three phosphate-rich bonds, or about 21 kcal, to build a 5-kcal bond.

The number of ribosomes per cell is of the order of about 10^7. Still, as the cell does not have an excess capacity for protein synthesis, any demand on it for increased output results in the production of more ribosomes.

RIBOSOMES AND THE NUCLEOLUS

Ribosomal RNA is characterized by a high proportion of GC bases. A similar base composition is found for the nucleolus, as organelle of the cell nucleus, varying in size and number in different species. During cell mitosis it disappears, reforming when the sister nuclei are reconstituted. It is always associated with a specific position on certain chromosomes, and this chromosomal locus is called the *nucleolar organizer.*

In the toad *Xenopus laevis* there is a mutant which lacks nucleoli. This condition is lethal at the tadpole stage. It was shown that embryos without nucleoli are unable to synthesize ribosomal RNA. In *Drosophila* the nucleolar organizer is on the X-chromosome. Rittosa and Spiegelman (1965) obtained strains with a deletion or a duplication of this locus. They then constructed strains with one, two, three, and four nucleolar organizers. From these strains they obtained purified DNA, and they checked for hybridization with ribosomal RNA, in increasing concentrations, to find out the amount needed to fully saturate the complementary DNA. The results are shown here in the original figure from that paper (Fig. 5-45).

Developing eggs of amphibians are quite large. Their nuclei reach a diameter of about 0.5 mm and are thus easy to isolate. In 1969, Miller and Beatty, investigating the nuclei of an amphibian, developed a method to obtain high resolution electron micrographs of their nucleoli. The appearance of the chromosomes at this stage led to their being called *lampbrush* chromosomes; they are extended, with large loops or material perpendicular to the main axis. These fibers contain material sensitive to DNAse, RNAse, and trypsin. Figure 5-46 is an electron micrograph of a segment along one of these loops. The bottom half of the figure shows RNA molecules being synthesized, and calls to mind the shape of a Christmas tree. The central axis is DNA; the fine grains along this axis are presumably RNA polymerases. The fibers extending from the axis can be removed by ribonuclease and trypsin, and have been shown to be ribosomal RNA precursor molecules coated with protein.

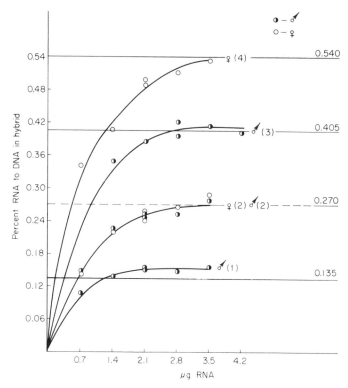

Fig. 5-45. Hybridization of DNA with RNA extracted from *Drosophila* strains containing one, two, three, and four nucleoles per nucleus. The number of nucleolar organizers present is indicated in parentheses. The numbers at the right are the assumed level of saturation. For a male with one organizer, 0.135 of the DNA corresponds to the ribosomal genes for the 18S and 28S RNA. (Courtesy of Rittosa and Spiegelman, *Proc. Nat. Acad. Sci.* 53:737, 1965.)

It has been shown that the nucleolus contains a large (45S) RNA molecule, which is the precursor of both 28S and 18S RNA. Special RNA polymerase and methylating enzymes exist in the nucleoli. During the maturation of this RNA inside the nucleolus, the precursor bases are partially methylated, and they cleave. The 5S RNA of ribosomes has a different and still unknown origin.

In 1970, Numora isolated pure proteins and RNA from the smaller ribosomal subunit of *E. coli.* When those components are mixed and incubated for some time, the subunit is reformed and is shown to be active. This reconstitution requires the simultaneous presence of the several proteins which must interact cooperatively. This is another good demonstration that subcellular structure is a thermodynamically spontaneous process and results from the primary structure of macromolecules.

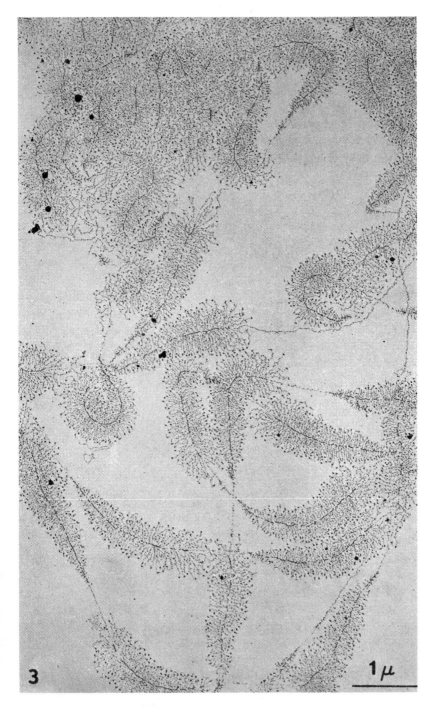

Fig. 5-46. Electron micrograph showing a segment of a lampbrush chromosome. RNA molecules being synthesized appear as perpendicular branches to the DNA molecule. (Courtesy of O. L. Miller and B. R. Beatty, *Science* 164:955, 1969.)

The factors involved in protein synthesis also occur in limited amounts, probably stoichiometrically with ribosomes. A recent finding of great medical interest is that the diphtheria toxin acts by inactivating one of the elongation factors. It functions as an enzyme, splitting NAD and transferring the adenine diphosphate ribose moiety to the factor, which becomes inactive.

BREAKING THE CODE

The information coded in the sequence of the mRNA bases is translated into a sequence of 20 different amino acids. The first attempt to devise a testable code came from the physicist George Gamow in 1954. If two of the four bases are combined, 4^2 combinations are obtained, which is less than the 20 codons needed. (A *codon* is defined as the unit coding for one amino acid.) Gamow came out with a different code that combined the four bases to give exactly 20 codons. He proposed that each amino acid was coded by four bases, placed as if in the corners of a diamond-shaped figure. Two of the bases were complementary pairs, belonging to two strands of the DNA molecule (Fig. 5-47).

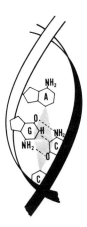

Fig. 5-47. Diamond code proposed by Gamow.

This proposal was made before it became known that the mRNA was a single-stranded molecule.

It is possible to combine the four nitrogen bases in many ways to develop codes for amino acids. In order to have twenty different codes, the bases must be combined in groups of three. These three base codons, or *triplets,* could then be arranged in a DNA chain in several possible ways. One way would be to separate the triplets with one or more bases, which would then be separate from the code and would act as a sort of genetic comma:

$$A\text{-}G\text{-}U\text{-}A\text{-}A\text{-}G\text{-}U\text{-}U\text{-}A\text{-}A\text{-}U\text{-}U\text{-}G. . .$$

$$AA_1 \quad , AA_2 \quad , AA_3$$

Of course, it would require fewer bases if the triplets could be connected together directly. This can be done if there is some reference point in the DNA to indicate the direction of the sequence:

$$A\text{-}G\text{-}U\text{-}G\text{-}U\text{-}U\text{-}U\text{-}U\text{-}G$$

$$AA_1 \quad AA_2 \quad AA_3$$

An even more economical arrangement would be an overlapping code in which each base would belong to two consecutive codons:

$$A\text{-}G\text{-}U\text{-}U\text{-}G$$

$$- AA_1 -$$
$$- AA_2 -$$
$$- AA_3 -$$

The overlapping code is the most economical but will not allow all random sequences of amino acids. In such a code, since one base belongs to up to three codons, a single mutation replacing one base should result in changes in more than one amino acid in the primary structure of a protein. As exemplified in abnormal hemoglobins, we always find one single amino acid replaced.

In 1961 Crick devised an experiment to test the genetic code. If we have a commaless code, and the reading starts at a specific point, the removal (or addition) of a single base would make the information after that point complete nonsense. He decided to use acridine to induce mutations into bacterial viruses. This planar compound interacts with DNA, interpolating itself between the paired bases (Fig. 5-48). This distorts the DNA molecule, and Crick proposed that it could result in deletion or insertion of one base. He isolated a number of mutants in a single gene and tried to recombine them. He was able to find two groups, which he named + and –. Recombinations between mutants of the same group did not reverse the gene to normal, but recombination of

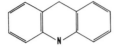

Fig. 5-48. Acriflavine.

a + and − did. He interpreted this as the result of combining a deletion with a nearby addition, thus restoring most of the information back to the original reading sequence.

normal	ATT	CGA	TCA	AGG	AAC	CCT	. . .
deletion	ATC	GAT	CAA	GGA	ACC	CC .	. . .
insertion	ATT	CGA	TTC	AAG	GAA	CCC	T . .
deletion plus insertion	ATC	GAT	TCA	AGG	AAC	CCT	. . .

He found that by introducing three, but not two or four, + mutations, he could make the gene operative, showing that the codon for one amino acid contained three bases.

The breakthrough came in 1961 when Nieremberg and Matthaei prepared a system from *E. coli,* including ribosomes and soluble components, that incorporated amino acids into proteins dependent on the addition of RNA as a messenger. By replacing the RNA with polyuridylic acid, they obtained the synthesis of polyphenylalanine, showing that the codon for this amino acid must be UUU. Using polynucleotide phosphorylase, Nieremberg and Ochoa's laboratories prepared a number of artificial RNAs with different proportions of bases and established the probable codons for many amino acids. In 1964, Nieremberg devised another method to check the code. A trinucleotide coding for one specific amino acid should be enough to bind the corresponding aminoacyl-tRNA to the ribosome. They measured the binding by using ^{14}C-aminoacyl-tRNA, and found that out of the 64 possible triplets, only three did not code for any amino acid. Of course, there is more than one triplet codon for the same amino acid, and the genetic code is therefore what is called *degenerate.*

Khorana's group developed methods for complete synthesis of DNA of a known sequence. Using this artificial DNA and DNA-dependent RNA polymerase, they prepared artificial messenger and used it to synthesize polypeptides.

Genetic Code

	Uracil		Cytosine		Adenine		Guanine	
Uracil	UUU	Phe	UCU	Ser	UAU	Tyr	UGU	Cys
	UUC	Phe	UCC	Ser	UAC	Tyr	UGC	Cys
	UUA	Leu	UCA	Ser	UAA	–	UGA	–
	UUG	Leu	UCG	Ser	UAG	–	UGG	Trp
Cytosine	CUU	Leu	CCU	Pro	CAU	His	CGU	Arg
	CUC	Leu	CCC	Pro	CAC	His	CGC	Arg
	CUA	Leu	CCA	Pro	CAA	Gln	CGA	Arg
	CUG	Leu	CCG	Pro	CAG	Gln	CGG	Arg
Adenine	AUU	Ile	ACU	Thr	AAU	Asn	AGU	Ser
	AUC	Ile	ACC	Thr	AAC	Asn	AGC	Ser
	AUA	Ile	ACA	Thr	AAA	Lys	AGA	Arg
	AUG	Met	ACG	Thr	AAG	Lys	AGG	Arg
Guanine	GUU	Val	GCU	Ala	GAU	Asp	GGU	Gly
	GUC	Val	GCC	Ala	GAC	Asp	GGC	Gly
	GUA	Val	GCA	Ala	GAA	Asp	GGA	Gly
	GUG	Val	GCG	Ala	GAG	Glu	GGG	Gly

Their analysis confirmed the code; the code is universal, from virus to man. Ochoa's group prepared oligonucleotides with the structure ApApAp . . . pApApApC, showing that this codes for LysLysLys . . . Asn, with the terminal amino group in the lysine and the terminal carboxyl group in the asparagine. Proteins are made from the free amino group end; thus, the messenger should read from 5′ to 3′.

The codon should correspond to an *anticodon* in the tRNA, and codon and anticodon should pair in antiparallel fashion, by formation of hydrogen bonds. Upon examining the codon, it is clear that whereas the pairing of the first two bases is well defined, the pairing of the third is less so. Crick, in his "wobble" hypothesis, proposed that the first and second bases would pair as expected according to the Watson-Crick model: a coupling with U on the anticodon and G coupling with anticodon C. He hypothesized that the third pairing would be less strict but would occur in a way predicted by ability to form stabilizing hydrogen bonds: either G or A in the codon would pair with U in the anticodon, and either U or C with G. Furthermore, we can expect that the anticodon could contain pseudouridine, which would pair with U in the codon; and inosine in the anticodon could pair with A, C, or U in the codon.

When the sequence of several tRNAs was deciphered, and the cloverleaf two-dimensional structure was written by pairing corresponding bases, it became clear that the anticodon was always in the same position. The anticodons of some tRNAs are

Ala	CGI
Tyr	AΨG
Ser	AGI
Phe	AAG
Val	CAI

Thus the 61 codons can be recognized by a much smaller number of tRNAs. Still, for some amino acids there are several tRNAs. In some cases, there are tRNAs specific for mitochondrial synthesis, a system independent of the nucleus.

In the specific case of Met-tRNA, there is one tRNA that is specific for the initiation of protein synthesis, and another for the insertion of methionine into the middle of the chain. Both respond to AUG, and it is not clear how the ribosome distinguishes one from the other. The nucleotide sequence of some messengers is at least partially known. It has been found that the sequence does not start with AUG, but that there are always a number of other nucleotides before this initiation signal. There is mounting evidence that the messenger is produced as a larger polynucleotide than the one needed for the coding, and that at one end it has a long sequence of poly A whose function is not known.

The three nonsense codons are signals for termination. They have been named ochre (UAA), amber (UAG), and umber (UGA); when they appear as a mutation in the middle of a messenger, they result in the termination of the chain and premature release of the growing polypeptide chain.

In at least one kind of mutation, a hemoglobin (called the *constant spring*) is produced that is longer than the normal hemoglobin, as if a nucleotide in the termination codon was changed to one coding for an amino acid, causing synthesis to continue beyond the normal termination point.

ERYTHROPOIETIN AND HEMOGLOBIN SYNTHESIS

Although hemoglobin synthesis is being actively studied, we still do not understand the fine details of its regulation. In the early embryonic stage, Gower's hemoglobin is synthesized in the blood islands of the yolk sac. All the cells differentiate at the same time, producing hemoglobin and developing into red cells, with the special hemoglobin chains present at that stage. Then the whole process comes to a halt. Some undifferentiated cells in the liver start to differentiate into red cell precursors. They produce alpha and gamma chains, which assemble as fetal hemoglobin. Much later in the development of the fetus, precursor cells appear in the bone marrow and spleen, where they begin to produce red cells with alpha and beta chains which assemble into the adult hemoglobin. Gamma chains are not made unless there is stress caused by a very severe anemia.

The synthesis of hemoglobin in a red cell takes about 100 hours. Hemoglobin mRNA seems to be a long-lasting molecule compared to many other messengers, which generally have very short lives. By preparing polysomes from reticulocytes and treating them with EDTA, it is possible to remove the ribosomes and separate the mRNA. The mRNA molecule has a sedimentation constant of 9S, and large-scale preparation and purification is possible. mRNA from one species can be mixed with ribosomes of a different species; the hemoglobin synthesized in this manner, as expected, corresponds to the species of the messenger.

Once we isolate mRNA, which can be made radioactive with labeled precursors, it would seem possible to locate the hemoglobin genes by hybridization with the chromosomes. This was possible with the genes that code for ribosomal RNA, since rRNA genes exist in a cluster of thousands of copies, but it is not the case with hemoglobin genes.

In recent years, a viral enzyme has been discovered with the ability to transcribe DNA from an RNA template. It is called *reverse transcriptase* and has been used to make DNA in vitro with hemoglobin mRNA as the template. The DNA produced is therefore identical to the hemoglobin gene.

It has been found that, during hemoglobin synthesis, some ribosomes make beta chains and others alpha chains. Although the amount of polysomes for each is different, equal amounts of alpha and beta chain are produced. The globin chains combine with heme and assemble in dimers and then in tetramers. If there is a shortage of heme, globin synthesis stops. If there is an excess of heme, it will block its own synthesis from succinate and glycine.

Injecting erythropoietin increases both the production of red cells and the amount of hemoglobin and red cell stroma (proteins that are recovered with membrane by high speed centrifugation of hemolyzed red cells) produced. This hormone acts also in vitro on explants of fetal liver or spleen maintained in culture. The synthesis of hemoglobin in a single cell does not increase, but the number of cells that differentiate to produce reticulocytes becomes larger. The hormone seems to act on a *stem* cell, which is the precursor of red cells, by inducing it to differentiate. By using x-rays (which kill cells in mitosis) and inhibitors of DNA synthesis, it was found that the hormone acts on cells that have undergone mitosis. Using radioactive precursors, it was shown that iron uptake increases four hours after hormone treatment, synthesis of stroma proteins in two hours, DNA synthesis in one hour, and RNA synthesis apparently as soon as 15 minutes after treatment.

Actinomycin, which inhibits the transcription of DNA into RNA, blocks the effect of the hormone. It seems that the hormone induces a sensitive cell to produce a new RNA, which causes this cell to begin differentiation. The cell will undergo four divisions, producing hemoglobin and stromal proteins, which develop into reticulocytes.

SELF-EVALUATION

1. Hemoglobins S, C, E, and Memphis result from the replacement of a single amino acid: glutamic acid by, respectively, valine, lysine, and glutamine. In each case, the glutamic acid codon is replaced by what codon (triplet)?

2. In a DNA molecule, according to the Watson-Crick model, bases pair by hydrogen bonds. Draw an A:T base pair and a G:C base pair as they would exist in a DNA molecule. Show the hydrogen bonds. It is a fact that DNA molecules with a higher G:C content melt at higher temperatures than DNA molecules with a lower G:C content. Why is this?

3. What amino acids can replace cysteine by changing a single nucleotide?

4. What are the genetic consequences of crossing-over and of sister exchange?

5. What is the difference between template and primer in DNA synthesis?

6. What is the role of the DNA repair enzymes?

7. What would happen if the two chains of DNA were transcribed in vivo into mRNA?

8. What supplies the energy requirements for protein synthesis?

9. What is the signal for the beginning of a message on the mRNA? For the end?

10. Where do actinomycin D, cycloheximide, and chloramphenicol act; and in order to what?

11. Where in the cell is there DNA replication? Where is there ribosomal RNA synthesis?

12. What happens when one nucleotide in a gene is deleted? How can the resulting effect be counteracted?

13. It was at one time considered a possibility that 18S ribosomal RNA resulted from cleavage of a 28S ribosomal RNA into two 18S rRNA particles. Devise an experiment to prove or disprove this theory. (Assume that the DNA genes which code for these ribosomal particles are available for your experiment.)

HEMOGLOBIN SYNTHESIS: A ROUND TABLE DISCUSSION

Prepare one of the following papers for discussion with students who have prepared others.

Grossbard, E., Terada, M., Dos, L., and Bank, A. Decrease of alpha globin messenger RNA activity associated with polyribosomes in alpha thalassaemia. *Nature (New Biology)* 241:209, 1973.

Gudon, J. B., Lane, D. C., Woodland, H. R., and Marbaix, G. Use of frog eggs and oocytes for the study of messenger RNA and its translation in living cells. *Nature* (Lond.) 233:177, 1971.

Kacian, D. L., Spiegelman, S., Bank, A., Terada, M., Metafora, S., Dow, L., and Marks, P. A. *In vitro* synthesis of DNA components of human genes for hemoglobin. *Nature (New Biology)* 235:167, 1972.

Mathews, M. B., Osborn, M., and Lingrel, J. Translation of globin messenger RNA in a heterologous cell-free system. *Nature* (Lond.) 233:206, 1971.

Nathan, D., Lodish, H., Kaan, Y. W., and Housman, D. Beta thalassemia and translation of globin messenger RNA. *Proc. Natl. Acad. Sci.* 68:2514, 1971.

Niehuis, A. W., Layckock, D. G., and Anderson, W. F. Translation of rabbit hemoglobin messenger RNA by thalassaemic and nonthalassaemic ribosomes. *Nature (New Biology)* 231:205, 1971.

Pemberton, R. E., Housman, D., Lodish, H., and Baglioni, C. Isolation of duck hemoglobin messenger RNA and its translation by rabbit reticulocyte cell-free system. *Nature (New Biology)* 235:99, 1972.

Ross, J., Ikawa, J., and Leder, D. Globin messenger RNA induction during erthroid differentiation of culture leukemia cells. *Proc. Natl. Acad. Sci.* 69:3620, 1972.

Terada, M., Cantor, L., Matafora, S., Rifkind, R. A., Bank, A., and Marks, P. Globin messenger RNA activity in erythroid precursor cells and the effect of erythropoietin. *Proc. Natl. Acad. Sci.* 69:3575, 1972.

Verman, I. M., Temple, G. F., Fan, H., and Baltimore. D. *In vitro* synthesis of DNA complementary to rabbit reticulocyte 10S RNA. *Nature (New Biology)* 235:163, 1972.

FURTHER READINGS

Bresnick, E., and Schwartz, A. *Functional Dynamics of the Cell.* New York: Academic, 1968.

Chargaff, E., and Davidson, J. N. *The Nucleic Acids.* 3 vols. New York: Academic, 1955–1960.

Davidson, J. N. *Biochemistry of Nucleic Acid.* New York: Wiley, 1969.

DeRobertis, E. D. P., Nowinski, W. W., and Saez, F. A. *Cell Biology.* Philadelphia: Saunders, 1970.

DuPraw, E. J. *Cell and Molecular Biology.* New York: Academic, 1968.

Hartman, P. E., and Suskin, S. R. *Gene Action.* 2nd ed. Englewood Cliffs, N.J.: Prentice-Hall, 1969.

Ingram, V. M. *Biosynthesis of Macromolecules.* New York: Benjamin, 1971.

Krantz, S. B., and Jacobson, L. O. *Erythropoietin and Regulation of Erythropoiesis.* Chicago: University of Chicago Press, 1970.

McCulloch, E. A. *Regulation of Hematopoiesis.* 2 vols. New York: Appleton-Century-Crofts, 1970.

Wolf, F. *Macromolecules, Structure and Function.* Englewoods Cliffs, N.J.: Prentice-Hall, 1971.

Collection of Classic Papers

Boyer, S. H. *Papers in Human Genetics.* Englewood Cliffs, N.J.: Prentice-Hall, 1963.

Gabrield, M. L., and Fogel, S. *Great Experiments in Biology.* Englewood Cliffs, N.J.: Prentice-Hall, 1955.

The Molecular Basis of Life. Readings from the *Scientific American.* San Francisco: Freeman, 1968.

Nishimura, S. *Selected Papers in Biochemistry.* Vols. 3, 5, and 6. Univ. Park. Press, 1971.

Peter, J. A. *Classical Papers in Genetics.* Englewood Cliffs, N.J.: Prentice-Hall, 1959.

Taylor, J. H. *Selected Papers on Molecular Genetics.* New York: Academic, 1965.

Zubay, G. *Papers in Biochemical Genetics.* New York: Academic, 1968.

ANNUAL REVIEWS

Annual Review of Biochemistry.

Annual Review of Genetics.

Progress in Nucleic Acid Research and Molecular Biology.

International Review of Cytology.

Advances in Cell and Molecular Biology.

Advances in Cell Biology.

6   Molecules to Population

STUDY GUIDE

Many of the problems related to the transmission of genetic traits and disease can be fully understood only in the context of the population as a whole. Population genetics is a very important field, having its beginnings in two papers early in this century, one by a mathematician and the other by a clinical doctor. Much progress in the theoretical aspects was achieved with the use of more sophisticated mathematics.

Man, in a society of constant change, has only recently begun to apply the field of population genetics to himself. Misunderstanding and intentional misinformation about population genetics has resulted in pseudoscientific bigotry and some innocuous, and other very dangerous, recommendations. Here can be seen the uncertain boundary between science and sociology.

You are expected to be able to

1. Explain the Hardy-Weinberg law and calculate the theoretical frequency of genes in equilibrium.

2. Explain the effect of social factors (migration, inbreeding, discrimination), selection, and mutation as they relate to changing gene frequencies.

3. Explain the role of selection for the heterozygote, which preserves deleterious recessive genes.

4. Describe the meaning of genetic load.

5. Discuss the role of eugeny in reducing the frequency of genetic diseases.

HARDY-WEINBERG LAW

If we wanted to conduct a genetic experiment with man, in the same manner as Mendel did with peas, we would take a couple representing a TT × tt grouping, where T (dominant) stands for the gene in which the capability to taste PTC is brought about, and t (recessive to T) for the allele for taste blindness, and move them to an island. (Isolation from all others is required.) In the first generation, we would expect only Tt children. These, through intermarriage, would give birth to 1/4 TT: 1/2 Tt: 1/4 tt groups. Therefore, in two generations the number of people who can taste PTC is 75 percent.

What would you expect in the third generation?

Let us start by checking the possible matings:

	1/4 TT	1/2 Tt	1/4 tt
1/4 TT	1/16	1/8	1/16
1/2 Tt	1/8	1/4	1/8
1/4 tt	1/16	1/8	1/16

These would produce the following offspring:

Mating	Frequency	Offspring TT	Offspring Tt	Offspring tt
TT × TT	1/16	1/16		
TT × Tt	1/4	1/8	1/8	
TT × tt	1/8		1/8	
Tt × Tt	1/4	1/16	1/8	1/16
Tt × tt	1/4		1/8	1/8
tt × tt	1/16			1/16
Sum	1	1/4 TT	1/2 Tt	1/4 tt

Thus we reach an equilibrium which will remain constant unless acted upon by other factors. Another way of looking at this setup is to calculate the gene frequency. In the initial couple there were half T genes and half t genes. The frequency of each gene was therefore 1/2. In the first generation, all the children were Tt, and the frequency of the two genes was maintained at the level of 1/2. The same frequency holds for the second generation, since there are 2 (1/4) + 1/2 = 1 T for every 1/2 + 2 (1/4) = 1 t.

If we start our human colony with three times more TT than tt, what would the genotype of the next generation be?

Mating	Frequency	Offspring		
		TT	Tt	tt
TT × TT	3/4 · 3/4	9/16		
TT × tt	2 · 3/4 · 1/4		6/16	
tt × tt	1/4 · 1/4			1/16
Sum	1	9/16	6/16	1/16

The gene frequency remains the same for this generation: for T, 2 (9/16) + 6/16 = 24/16; and for t, 6/16 + 2/16 = 8/16, which gives us the ratio T:t = 3:1. Hardy and Weinberg independently concluded in 1908 that the gene frequency of a population undergoing random mating will remain constant.

We can now generalize, using the letter p to mean the frequency of the gene T, and the letter q to mean the frequency of the gene t (assuming there are only two alleles), with $p + g = 1$ (the total of the two alleles). Now, when this population reaches equilibrium, the proportion of TT depends on the chances of the two genes T being in the same individual, that is, $p \times p = p^2$. We will then get the following ratios: p^2 TT : 2 pq Tt : q^2 tt (Fig. 6-1).

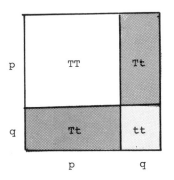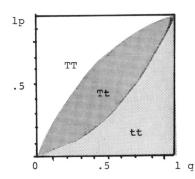

Fig. 6-1. Proportion of genotypes in a population in equilibrium according to the Hardy-Weinberg law.

In relation to capacity to taste PTC, marriage is random. No man or woman knows the phenotype of his or her possible mate. This is not true in the case of height, for example; men very frequently marry shorter women. We can test the random mating in relation to PTC tasting to see if it fulfills the known equilibrium. Use the data obtained earlier by your colleagues (Chapter 4) (by eliminating blood relatives, you are more certain of having a random sample of the population). Using the frequency of the nontasters, you can calculate q. The frequency of tasters is $p^2 + 2\,pq$. From the value of q, one can calculate p, which has to be $1 - q$.

Another way of testing the Hardy-Weinberg equilibrium is to compare the ratio of types of mating and the resulting offspring with expected values. In Table 6-1 you will find the expected results. Compile the data from the

Table 6-1. Frequency of Mating Types and Offspring Ratios

Mating	Genotype	Frequency	Offspring TT	Tt	tt	Total
taster	$TT \times TT$	p^4	p^4	0	0	
$\times$						
taster	$TT \times Tt$	$4p^3q$	$2p^3q$	$2p^3q$	0	
	$Tt \times Tt$	$4p^2q^2$	p^2q^2	$2p^2q2$	p^2q^2	
		$p^2(1+q)$	p^2	$2p^2q$	p^2q^2	$(q/1+q)^2$
taster	$TT \times tt$	$2p^2q^2$	0	$2p^2q^2$	0	
$\times$						
nontaster	$Tt \times tt$	$4pq^3$	0	$2pq^3$	$2pq^3$	
		$2pq^2(1+q)$	0	$2pq^2$	$2pq^3$	$q/1+q$
nontaster $\times$ nontaster	$tt \times tt$	q^4	0	0	q^4	all

entire set of pedigrees and check to see if the pedigrees represent a real random mating population. Remember that the concentration of PTC used in the testing assures that about 98 percent of the tasters will be found. Some who test as nontasters, however, will be able to detect PTC at higher concentrations.

The frequency of cases with thalassemia is about one per million. Using the Hardy-Weinberg law, we can say that the frequency of the gene for thalassemia is the square root of 1/1,000,000, or 1/1,000. From this figure and the fact that the frequency of carriers is 2pq, we can calculate this frequency to be $2(999/1,000) (1/1,000) \cong 1/500$. Mating between carriers would be about $1/500 \times 1/500$, a probability of 1/250,000.

Is man a population in equilibrium?

The primitive human society has always consisted of small isolated groups. In a small population the equilibrium is related, to a large extent, to chance. The premature death of a single individual may eliminate a rare gene. Also, since the number of children from one couple is small, not all the genes may be transmitted to the next generation. Thus, a couple with only sons would have lost the father's X-chromosome. It is still possible to detect the effect of chance in genetics (referred to as *genetic drift*) in some rare isolated populations. This is true of a particular religious group in Pennsylvania, the Older Order of Amish, founded in 1774 by a single couple. They must have had a rare gene which resulted in dwarfism and extra digits. Today about half the total number of cases of this rare anomaly come from that group. About 13 percent of the 8,000 members of the group carry this gene.

Lack of genetic exchange through sociocultural or geographical isolation has resulted in groups with different gene frequencies. It is this fact that characterizes a race. A race is determined by a group attribute that has a different average gene frequency from the frequency it has in other groups.

This variety provided the raw material for the rise of man as a species. The more man was able to control his environment, the less his survival depended on genetic adaptation to the environment. With the Industrial Revolution came the invention of transportation. This led to large migratory movements and the creation of dense population areas. Random marriage became more common. Each individual has a wider choice today as far as finding a mate is concerned.

Table 6-2, showing the frequency of the gene for PTC taste-blindness, illustrates this point. Considerable differences exist between populations from different continents. The American continents illustrate a move toward a single mating population. Compared to the original African Negro, the Brazilian Negro shows about half of a white genetic pool. In the United States the northern Negro has about 30 percent white-originated genes. This proportion is much higher in the South.

CONSANGUINITY

The chance that a child from a first-cousin marriage will inherit a particular gene twice is 1/64. Because in the two parents there are four alleles to each

Table 6-2. Frequency of the PTC Taste-Blindness Gene

Europe		Asia-Oceania	
Sweden	0.57	China	0.33
Denmark	0.58	Japan	0.34
Finland	0.54	Australoids	0.70
Norway	0.55		
England	0.57	Africa	
Spain	0.50		
Portugal	0.49	Egypt	0.49
Italy	0.49	Occidental Africa	0.16
		Bantus	0.20
Brazil			
		USA	
Whites	0.50		
Indians	0.11	White	0.54
Ashkenazi Jews	0.53	Negroes (Ohio)	0.30
Japanese	0.36	Negroes (Alabama)	0.48
Negroes	0.36	Indians	0.36

gene, the chance of a child's being a homozygote for any one of the genes is $1/64 \times 4 = 1/16$. (See Figure 6-2.) (This number is called the *inbreeding coefficient;* its value differs according to the grade of relatedness.)

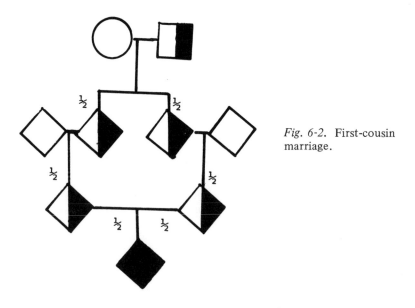

Fig. 6-2. First-cousin marriage.

The chance for a normal child, from a first-cousin marriage, to be heterozygous for the deleterious gene is $15/16$. However, this number goes down very fast as the number of abnormal genes increases. This is because the chance for heterozygosis is $(15/16)^n$. Man has many abnormal genes, and, therefore, about one-half to two-thirds of all cases of genetic diseases appear among offspring of first-cousin marriages.

Even before man understood the mechanism of genetic transmission, rules had been established to prevent consanguinity. All major religions have rules prohibiting incest. Taboos and prohibitions existed in every primitive society. (In Persian law, even homosexual relationships were taken into account in avoiding this consanguinity.) The only groups that disregarded those social and religious rules were the royal families. Two Egyptian dynasties (that which included Tutankhamon and that which included Cleopatra) had sister-brother and uncle-niece marriages. Oedipus's story of mother-son marriage probably originated from the history of the eighteenth Egyptian dynasty. Inbreeding led to a lack of male offspring, total sterility, and other handicaps that resulted in the extinction of that particular group.

Assuming that there is one generation every 25 years, i.e., about 40 per millenium, any one individual must have had 2^{40} (1,099,511,627,766) ancestors. A millenium ago, earth's population was about 200 million. This shows the extent of inbreeding which took place. First-cousin marriages have been frequently recorded, especially by the Catholic Church, which requires special authorization for a wedding of this type. Vatican data shows an increase of inbreeding between 1850 and 1900 when the first industrial districts arose, but it has been falling steadily since. This is the result of increasing population density in cities, decrease of family size, and larger human mobility.

First-cousin marriages generally account for about 0.5 to 1 percent of the marriages in developed countries. In some countries it is much higher, reaching 5.5 percent in Japan and 8.6 percent in India, due to their social structure.

Brazil is probably one of the better-studied countries in this respect. In less developed regions, first-cousin marriages reach 4 to 5 percent, but these drop to about 1 percent in the south. From the frequency of the first-cousin marriages, one can calculate the size of the mating population, using mathematical formulas and models developed by Dahlberg. In the region of São Paulo, the fastest growing city in the world, about 40 percent of all marriages in the eighteenth century were consanguineous. In the first half of the last century only 7 percent were first-cousin marriages. These represent a mating isolate on the order of 450. The number of consanguineous marriages dropped in 1963 to 0.85 percent, representing an isolate of about 3,000. This means that 150 years ago, an individual in São Paulo could choose a mate from among 225 different people.

In 1963, living in a city of about 3 million, he has a choice among about 1,500 of the opposite sex.

For a gene with a frequency of 0.01 (according to the Hardy-Weinberg law) in a random mating population, we expect 0.01^2 or 1/10,000 homozygotes. In the case of first-cousin marriages, the number of homozygotes is about six times larger. Inbreeding results in an increase of homozygosis (Fig. 6-3).

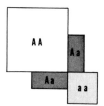

Fig. 6-3. Effect of consanguinity on the proportion of genotypes in a population in equilibrium.

SELECTION

Another factor that disturbs the equilibrium predicted by the Hardy-Weinberg law is selection. Hardy-Weinberg equilibrium presupposes not just random mating but also equal chances of perpetuation through descendants for all genotypes.

From the point of view of population genetics, it does not make much difference if a certain genotype leads to early death, stillbirth, or sterility. The result is the same: *genetic death,* or lack of transmission of genes to the next generation. Furthermore, a decrease in fertility, even by a small fraction of the average number of children per couple, is as significant in this respect as a genetic death. Thus genetic death occurs through lack of transmission of the genes through continuing generations, not necessarily by actual death of an individual carrying the gene.

If a gene is dominant and causes total infertility, like chondrodystrophic dwarfism, (an abnormality in the growth of the bones of limbs), it is eliminated in one generation. If it is dominant but decreases fertility only by one-half, it takes over ten generations for the genes to be eliminated (Fig. 6-4). With a 1 percent selection rate, i.e., a small fertility handicap, the gene would last much longer. (If it were a common gene, present in 99 percent of a population, it would take 4,000 generations to drop to one-half, about 7,000 generations to fall to one-tenth, and 90,000 generations until it goes down to 0.1 percent.)

If the gene involved in the selection process is recessive, the effectiveness of selection is much smaller. For a gene with a frequency of 0.1, there are 0.01

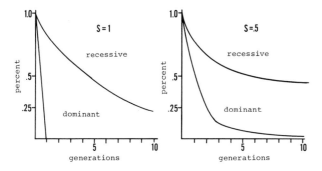

Fig. 6-4. Effect of selection on dominant and recessive traits.

homozygotes and 0.18 heterozygotes. Even a fully efficient selection would act slowly. This is because it does not reduce the transmission of the genes from one generation to the next from the large number of heterozygotes.

It is possible that the heterozygote of a deleterious recessive gene would have its fitness somewhat diminished. In this case the selection would also act to a smaller degree on the heterozygotes.

A not uncommon phenomenon is increase of fitness of the heterozygote (Fig. 6-5). The increase of height in recent years has been attributed to larger outbreeding. In plants, inbreeding results in smaller yields. Hybrid corn is an example of a maximization by heterozygosis.

Fig. 6-5. Effect of the increased fitness of the heterozygote in the proportion of genotypes in a population in equilibrium

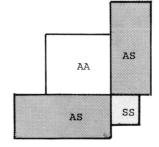

A very important discovery was the association of malaria with hemoglobin defects. It was found that hemoglobins S and C, thalassemias, and primaquine anemias occur in Asia, Africa, southern Europe, and the Mediterranean basin, where malaria is common. Malaria occurs through the action of a parasite, which has part of its cycle inside the red cells. It was found, as will be seen in the paper at the end of this chapter, that there were fewer patients with malaria among the heterozygotes for sickle cell anemia or C hemoglobin, and that among those that did exist, fewer presented the cerebral form and died from it. Heterozygotes are less susceptible to experimental malaria.

This relative immunity to malaria resulted in a selection in favor of the heterozygote, because the homozygote of the abnormal S hemoglobin has sickle cell anemia, whereas the normal homozygote is more susceptible to malaria. The frequency of the S gene rose to as high as 20 percent in some regions.

Hemoglobin C has a frequency of about 27 percent in West Africa, it can be expected to compete favorably with hemoglobin S because it protects against malaria in the heterozygote form, and, on the other hand, does not produce severe anemia in the homozygote.

The selection pattern changes as conditions change. This is true in the case of Negroes living in malaria-free areas of the American continent. Now AA and AS individuals have the same longevity, selection being made only against the SS types. The same occurs in the Mediterranean region, where malaria is now under control thanks to the introduction of DDT.

Civilization led to relaxation of selection. Myopia was a severe handicap for the primitive hunting man, but is no handicap in the modern world. Babies with cleft palates or intestinal obstructions, who would normally die soon after birth, are now being rescued and their defects corrected through surgery. Diabetes is more common today than it was forty years ago, when it was considered lethal because insulin was not available.

It has been found that thyroid deficiency is more common among nontasters of PTC. Do you feel that the data you have studied shows any deviation due to selection?

Selection should continuously decrease the frequency of genes that result in physically unfit specimens. True, it is a very slow process for a rare recessive gene, but for the dominant gene with a selection rate of 1, it would take only one generation.

But such genes do not disappear. An example is retinoblastoma, a retinal tumor which is transmitted on a dominant gene. It results in death before reproduction age. Yet between 1936 and 1945, 49 new cases appeared in Michigan in a sample of 1 million children. Thus we must assume that new cases appear with a frequency of about 2×10^{-5}, through the transformation of the normal allele in the retinoblastoma gene. This transformation process is called *mutation.*

Most mutations occurring in a population adapted to its environment must be deleterious, and are normally eliminated by selection. Equilibrium is thus established only when mutation and selection rates are equal.

It is possible to estimate the mutation rate through the selection rate, that is, by comparing the (reduced) number of offspring that carry a mutated gene to those carrying a normal allele. This, however, is difficult to assess in man because of his limited offspring and because about 30 percent of fertilized eggs do not result in childbirth.

Data available suggest that the mutation rate is around 1×10^{-5} to 4×10^{-5}. When much larger numbers are found, as in the case of deaf-mutism, it means presumably that there are several genes that result in the same phenotype. It is easy to imagine several different defects leading to deaf-mutism.

GENETIC LOAD

When we compare the families of first-cousin couples with nonrelated couples living in the same environment and conditions, we find a 5 percent increase in child mortality in the former group. We must assume this to be the effect of deleterious genes, referring to the 1 chance in 64 of homozygosis in the first-cousin couples' offspring. This represents $64 \times .05$, or 3.2, recessive lethal genes present if we assume that this 5 percent increase in infant mortality is due to recessive lethal genes.

If we assume (1) that mutation rate is about 2×10^{-5} and (2) that man has about 20,000 genes, we can expect 40 percent of the human population to carry a new mutation. Each new mutation must be removed by selection to reestablish equilibrium. This genetic death may not necessarily represent a cadaver or a suffering, handicapped person. It may mean simple sterility or lower fertility that may not even be noticeable because of the present trend toward smaller families. Still, about 11 births per thousand consist of abnormal children, which gives a mortality of about 30 percent in living offspring.

This, then, is the cost of mutation, a *mutational load* that is essential for providing the species with genetic variability, essential for adaptation and evolution.

Another type of load arises from balanced polymorphism, in which heterozygotes are more fitted for survival than homozygotes. On mating homozygotes with apparently low fitness, we get what is called a *segregational load*. It has been estimated, through experiments with drosophila, that about 20 percent of all genes are heterozygous in nature.

Studies on human populations estimate that an average load is about 4 lethal equivalents per person. A lethal equivalent or *lethon* would cause, on an average, one genetic death. These estimates equate two semilethal genes (i.e., s = 0.5) with one fully lethal gene.

EUGENY

If we assume the presence of a rare recessive gene, with a frequency of 1/1,000, in a population of a million persons, and assume a birth rate of about 50,000 per year, we would have the following:

Genotype	Frequency		Persons
Double recessive carriers	q^2	10^{-6}	1
Heterozygotes	2pq	.002	2,000
New mutants		2×10^{-5}	20

It is obvious that if the homozygotes for this disease were prevented from having offspring , this would not affect the presence of the gene in the population.

Negative eugeny — enforcing reproduction restriction against carriers of deleterious genes — was a fashionable idea with the establishment of Mendelian genetics around the beginning of this century. However, it was mixed with bigotry, pseudoscientific politics, and religious bias. It imposed compulsory sterilization and even euthanasia. With the development of mathematical foundations of population genetics and a better knowledge of human genetics, the idea was abandoned. To prevent carriers of deleterious genes from reproducing would deny 99 percent of the population the right to have children. Dominant genes and sex-linked genes which do not impair reproduction but are deleterious are the only instances in which negative eugeny has any meaning. And in this case genetic counseling remains the accepted procedure.

Many deleterious genetic traits are transmitted as recessive genes. Today we can distinguish a heterozygote from the normal homozygous person for about two dozen hereditary diseases, thus providing more data for genetic counseling.

An important development is the possibility of obtaining embryonic cells by puncturing the amniotic cavity. Those cells can be cultivated and used to detect several hereditary diseases. This provides the parents with advance information which may help in decisions regarding the pregnancy.

The present trend toward smaller families, dense populations, mobility, social change, and increasing random mating is leading to more heterozygosis. One can therefore expect a decrease in recessive genetic diseases through the dissemination of the genes for them. This will result in a future of homozygosis and selection, leading to the same number of genetic deaths, but more dilute in intensity. We will also have a lower rate of birth defects found in isolates.

Positive eugeny (selecting who should breed) has been proposed by a number of eminent scientists — Serebrovsky in Russia, Muller in the United States, and Julian Huxley in England. The control of the genetic pool of man by man seems an obvious step. Man has controlled, without really understanding, the genetic pool of plants and animals since the dawn of civilization. Goals in applied plant and animal selection are quite simple (e.g., increased milk production, higher corn yields, and resistance to rust). But it is very difficult to judge the number of different qualities a man should have, both in terms of his present way of living and, more important, in terms of a future civilization whose requirements and demands we cannot foresee. Engineering for a supposed optimum may represent disaster. This has occurred recently in the case of some farm crops. All the farmers in one large region used the seeds of a particularly productive strain, which was destroyed by an unexpected parasite. Variability is the source of adaptation and evolution of a species.

SELF-EVALUATION

1. State the conditions and consequences of the Hardy-Weinberg law.

2. In a population of 100,000, there are 16,000 persons with a genetic disease which is transmitted by a recessive gene. If those persons are not allowed to have children, what would be the frequency of persons with this disease in the next generation?

3. A population living in a certain area was studied for a hereditary characteristic and was found not to be in equilibrium. State as many hypotheses as you can to explain this.

4. Negative eugeny can decrease the frequency of
   a. recessive genes.
   b. dominant genes.
   c. sex-linked genes.

PROTECTION AFFORDED BY SICKLE-CELL TRAIT AGAINST SUBTERTIAN MALARIAL INFECTION†

A. C. Allison

The aetiology of sickle-cell anaemia presents an outstanding problem common to both genetics and medicine. It is now universally accepted that the sickle-cell anomaly is caused by a single mutant gene which is responsible for the production of a type of haemoglobin differing in several important respects from normal adult haemoglobin (Pauling *et al.*, 1949; Perutz and Mitchison, 1950). Carriers of the sickle-cell trait who are heterozygous for the sickle-cell gene have a mixture of this relatively insoluble haemoglobin and normal haemoglobin; hence their erythrocytes do not sickle *in vivo,* whereas some at least of the homozygotes, who have a much greater proportion of sickle-cell haemoglobin, have sickle cells in the circulating blood, with inevitable haemolysis and a severe, often fatal, haemolytic anaemia. There is also a much smaller group of sickle-cell anaemia patients who are heterozygous for the sickle-cell gene as well as for some other hereditary abnormality of haemoglobin synthesis (Neel, 1952).

It is thus possible to approach the problem from the clinical or the genetical side. From the clinical point of view it is important to distinguish between carriers of the sickle-cell trait who show no other haematological abnormalities and patients with sickle-cell anaemia, who have a haemolytic disease which can reasonably be attributed to sickling of the erythrocytes. From the genetical point of view the main distinction is to be drawn between those who are homozygous and those who are heterozygous for the sickle-cell gene. In the great majority of instances two classifications coincide—that is, most individuals with the sickle-cell trait are heterozygous and most cases of sickle-cell anaemia, in Africa at least, are homozygous for the sickle-cell gene.

The sickle-cell trait is remarkably common in some parts of the world. Among many African Negro tribes 20% or more of the total population have the trait, and frequencies of 40% have been found in several African tribes (Lehmann and Raper, 1949; Allison, 1954). In parts of Greece frequencies of 17% have been described (Choremis *et al.*, 1953), and as many as 30% of the population in Indian aboriginal groups are affected (Lehmann and Cutbush, 1952).

Wherever the sickle-cell trait is known to occur sickle-cell anaemia

† This investigation was made possible by a grant received from the Colonial Office at the recommendation of the Colonial Medical Research Committee. Acknowledgment is made to the Directors of Medical Services, Kenya and Uganda, to Dr. E. J. Foley, Nairobi, to the staff of the Mulago Hospital, Kampala, and to the volunteers for their kind cooperation. To Dr. G. I. Robertson, Nairobi, a special debt of gratitude is due for constant help and advice. Drs. A. E. Mourant, R. G. Macfarlane, and A. H. T. Robb-Smith read the manuscript and made valuable comments and suggestions.

will also be found. For a time it was thought by some workers that sickle-cell anaemia was rare among African Negroes, but so many cases have been described during the past few years that this view is no longer tenable (Lambotte-Legrand and Lambotte-Legrand, 1951; Foy *et al.*,1951; Edington, 1953; Vandepitte and Louis, 1953).

The main problem can be stated briefly: how can the sickle-cell gene be maintained at such a high frequency among so many peoples in spite of the constant elimination of these genes through deaths from the anaemia? Since most sickle-cell anaemia subjects are homozygotes, the failure of each one to reproduce usually means the loss of two sickle-cell genes in every generation. It can be estimated that for the lost genes to be replaced by recurrent mutation so as to leave a balanced state, assuming that the sickle-cell trait—that is, the heterozygous condition—is neutral from the point of view of natural selection, it would be necessary to have a mutation rate of the order of 10^{-1}. This is about 3,000 times greater than naturally occurring mutation rates calculated for man and, with rare exceptions, in many other animals — 3.2×10^{-5} in the case of haemophilia (Haldane, 1947). A mutation rate of this order of magnitude can reasonably be excluded as an explanation of the remarkably high frequencies of the sickle-cell trait observed in Africa and elsewhere.

POSSIBILITY OF SELECTIVE ADVANTAGE

Of the other explanations which can be advanced to meet the situation, one has received little attention: the possibility that individuals with the sickle-cell trait might under certain conditions have a selective advantage over those without the trait. It was stated for many years that the sickle-cell trait was in itself a cause of morbidity, but this belief seems to have been based upon unsatisfactory criteria for distinguishing the trait from sickle-cell anaemia. The current view is that the sickle-cell trait is devoid of selective value. Henderson and Thornell (1946) found that in American Negro air cadets who had passed a searching physical examination the incidence of the sickle-cell trait was the same as in the general Negro population of the United States. Lehmann and Milne (1949) were unable to discover any correlation between haemoglobin levels and the presence or absence of the sickle-cell trait in Uganda Africans. And Humphreys (1952) could find no evidence that the sickle-cell trait was responsible for any morbidity in Nigerian soldiers.

However, during the course of field work undertaken in Africa in 1949 I was led to question the view that the sickle-cell trait is neutral from the point of view of natural selection and to reconsider the possibility that it is associated with a selective advantage. I noted then that the incidence of the sickle-cell trait was higher in regions where malaria was prevalent than elsewhere. The figures presented by Lehmann and Raper (1949) for the frequency of the sickle-cell trait in different parts of Uganda lent some support to this view, as did the published reports from elsewhere. Thus the trait is fairly common in parts of Italy and Greece, but rare in other European countries; in Greece the trait attains its highest frequencies in areas which are conspicuously malarious (Choremis *et al.*, 1951).

RELATION BETWEEN MALARIA AND SICKLE-CELL TRAIT

Other reports appeared suggesting more directly that there might be a relationship between malaria and the sickle-cell trait. Beet (1946) had observed that in a group of 102 sicklers from the Balovale district of Northern Rhodesia only 10 (9.8%) had blood slides showing malaria parasites, whereas in a comparable group of 491 non-sicklers 75 (15.3%) had malaria parasites. The difference in incidence of malaria in the two groups is statistically highly significant ($x^2 = 19.349$ for 1 d.f.);[1] hence Beet's figures imply strongly that malaria is less frequent among individuals with the sickle-cell trait than among those without the trait. The difference in malarial susceptibility between sicklers and others seemed to be most pronounced at the time of the year when malaria transmission was lowest.

Later in the Fort Jameson district of Northern Rhodesia, Beet (1947) found that the same difference was present, although it was much less pronounced. Of, 1,019 non-sicklers, 312 (30.6%) had blood slides with malaria parasites, whereas of 149 sicklers 42 (28.2%) showed malaria parasites. This difference is not statistically significant. However, among the sicklers from Fort Jameson enlarged spleens were less common than among non-sicklers. In a series of 569 individuals there were 87 with the sickle-cell trait; 24 (27.9%) of these had palpable spleens, as compared with 188 (39.0%) with splenomegaly out of 482 non-sicklers. This difference is again statistically significant ($x^2 = 4.11$ for 1 d.f.). Beet concluded that Africans with the sickle-cell trait were probably liable to recurrent attacks of thrombosis, with resultant shrinkage of the spleen.

Brain (1952a), also working in Rhodesia, confirmed Beet's observation that the spleen is palpable in a much lower proportion of sicklers than of non-sicklers; he went on to suggest that the finding might be explained by diminished susceptibility to malaria on the part of the sicklers. Moreover, Brain (1952b) compared the proportion of hospitalized cases in groups of African mine-workers with and without the sickle-cell trait. He found that the sicklers actually spent less time in hospital, on an average, than did the control group of non-sicklers. The incidence of malaria and pyrexias of unknown origin was much lower in the group with sickle cells.

It became imperative, then, to ascertain by more direct methods of investigation whether sickle cells can afford some degree of protection against malarial infection, thereby conferring a selective advantage on possessors of the sickle-cell trait in regions where malaria is hyperendemic. An opportunity to do this came during the course of a visit to East Africa in 1953.

INCIDENCE OF MALARIAL PARASITAEMIA IN AFRICAN CHILDREN WITH AND WITHOUT THE SICKLE-CELL TRAIT

The observations of Beet and of Brain on differences in parasite rates and spleen rates are open to criticism because the populations were heterogeneous and were drawn from relatively wide areas. It was decided, therefore, to carry out similar tests on a relatively small circumscribed community, where all those under observation belong to a single tribe. Children were chosen rather than adults as subjects for the observations so as to minimize the effect of acquired immunity to malaria. The recorded incidence of parasitaemia in a group of 290 Ganda children, aged 5 months to 5 years, from the area surrounding

---

[1] These and other statistics in this paper are my own, using available figures.

Table 1.

	With parasitaemia	Without parasitaemia	Total
Sicklers........	12 (27.9%)	31 (72.1%)	43
Non-sicklers	113 (45.7%)	134 (53.3%)	247

Kampala (excluding the non-malarious township) is presented in Table 1.

The presence of sickling was demonstrated by chemical reduction of blood with isotonic sodium metabisulphite (Daland and Castle, 1948). Fresh reducing solutions were made up daily.

It is apparent that the incidence of parasitaemia is lower in the sickle-cell group than in the group without sickle cells. The difference is statistically significant (x^2 = 5.1 for 1 d.f.). In order to test as many families as possible only one child was taken from each family. There is no reason to suppose that these groups are not comparable, apart from the presence or absence of the sickle-cell trait.

The parasite density in the two groups also differed: of 12 sicklers with malaria, 8 (66.7%) had only slight parasitaemia (group 1 on an arbitrary rating), while 4 (33.3%) had a moderate parasitaemia (group 2). Of the 113 non-sicklers with malaria, 34% had slight parasitaemia (group 1), the parasite density in the remainder being moderate or severe (group 2 or 3).

It may be noted, incidentally, that of the four cases in the sickle-cell group with moderate parasitaemia three had *P. malariae,* even though this species is much less common than *P. falciparum* around Kampala. It seems possible from these and other observations that the protection afforded by the sickle-cell trait is more effective against *P. falciparum* than against other species of plasmodia, but much further work is necessary to decide the point.

These results suggest that African children with the sickle-cell trait have malaria less frequently or for shorter periods, and perhaps also less severely, than children without the trait. Further evidence regarding the protective action of the sickle-cell trait could be obtained only by direct observation on the course of artificially induced malarial infection in volunteers.

PROGRESS OF MALARIAL INFECTION IN ADULT AFRICANS WITH AND WITHOUT THE SICKLE-CELL TRAIT

Fifteen Luo with the trait and 15 Luo without the trait were accepted for this investigation. All the volunteers were adult males who had been away from a malarious environment for at least 18 months. The two groups were of a similar age and appeared to be strictly comparable apart from the presence or absence of the sickle-cell trait. Two strains of *P. falciparum* were used—one originally isolated in Malaya and one from near Mombasa, Kenya; in Table II these are marked with the subscripts 1 and 2 respectively. The infection was introduced by subinoculation with 15 ml. of blood containing a large number of trophozoites (B in the table) or by biting with heavily infected *Anopheles gambiae* (M in the table). At least 3 out of the 10 mosquitoes applied had bitten each individual, and the presence of sporozoites was confirmed by dissection of the mosquitoes.

The cases were followed for 40 days. Parasite counts for each case were made by comparison with the number of leucocytes in 200 oil-immersion fields of thick films, the absolute leucocyte counts being checked at intervals. The abbreviated results of these counts are shown in Table II. In the few cases in which parasitaemia was pronounced and the symptoms were relatively severe the progress of the disease was arrested. At the end of the period of observation in every case a pro-longed course of antimalarial chemotherapy was given.

DISCUSSION

It is apparent that the infection has become established in 14 cases without the sickle-cell trait. The parasitaemia is relatively light, how-ever, when compared with that observed in non-immune populations—for example, the Africans described by Thomas *et al.* (1953). This is to be expected: the Luo come from a part of the country where malaria is hyperendemic, and they have acquired a considerable immunity to malarial infection in childhood. This factor makes the interpretation of the observations rather more difficult; however, it could not be avoided, since all the East African tribes who have high sickling rates come from malarious areas, and the acquired immunity should operate with equal force in the groups with and without sickle-cells. The ac-quired immunity was actually an advantage, since the symptoms were mild and the chances of complication very slight.

In the group with sickle cells, on the other hand, the malaria parasites have obviously had great difficulty in establishing themselves, in spite of repeated artificial infection. Only two of the cases show parasites, and the parasite counts in these cases are comparatively low. The striking difference in the progress of malarial infection in the two groups is taken as evidence that the abnormal erythrocytes in individuals with the sickle-cell trait are less easily parasitized than are normal erythrocytes.

It can therefore be concluded that individuals with the sickle-cell trait will, in all probability suffer from malaria less often and less severely than those without the trait. Hence in areas where malaria is hyperendemic children having the trait will tend to survive, while some children without the trait are eliminated before they acquire a solid immunity to malarial infection. The protection against malaria might also increase the fertility of possessors of the trait. The proportion of individuals with sickle cells in any population, then, will be the result of a balance between two factors; the severity of malaria, which will tend to increase the frequency of the gene, and the rate of elimination of the sickle-cell genes in individuals dying of sickle-cell anaemia. Or, genetically speaking, this is a balanced polymorphism where the heterozygote has an advantage over either homozygote.

The incidence of the trait in East Africa has recently been investigated in detail (Allison, 1954), and found to vary in accordance with the above hypothesis. High frequencies are observed among the tribes living in regions where malaria is hyperendemic (for example, around Lake Vic-toria and in the Eastern Coastal Belt), whereas low frequencies occur consistently in the malaria-free or epidemic zones (for example, the Kigezi district of Uganda; the Kenya Highlands; and the Kilimanjaro, Mount Meru, and Usumbara regions of Tanganyika). This difference is

Table II.

No.	Mode of infection and strain	Day after infection																
		8	10	12	14	16	18	20	22	24	26	28	30	32	34	36	38	40
		Luo with no sickle-cells																
1	M_2 B_1	0.03	—	0.07	2.5	5.0	2.5	5.0	1.2	0.4	0.02	0.01	—	—	0.1	0.01	0.01	ST
2	M_2 B_1	—	—	—	—	—	—	—	0.03	0.13	0.41	5.0	2.5	1.25	1.67	0.03	—	ST
3	M_2 B_1	—	—	—	—	0.02	0.02	0.5	0.1	0.02	0.20	1.0	1.0	0.83	0.25	0.2	5.0	2.0 S
4	M_2 B_1	—	5.0	10.0	10.0	0.05	1.0	1.67	0.83	0.12	0.2	0.25	1.0	1.0	0.03	0.17	—	ST
5	M_2 B_2	0.02	—	—	—	1.0	0.1	0.01	0.25	0.05	0.07	—	1.2	—	—	—	—	ST
6	B_1	—	—	—	—	15.0	50.0	ST	ST	—	—	—	—	—	—	—	—	—
7	B_2	—	—	0.13	5.0	1.67	0.33	—	—	—	—	—	—	—	—	—	—	—
8	B_1	—	—	—	—	5.0	—	0.1	0.5	ST	—	—	—	—	—	—	—	—
9	B_2	—	—	—	—	—	—	0.05	0.05	2.5	—	1.0	0.1	2.5	10.0	5.0	0.5	ST
10	B_1	—	0.05	—	—	—	—	0.2	—	—	—	0.67	—	0.1	0.05	5.0	5.0	ST
11	B_2	—	—	0.3	0.3	0.3	0.1	0.2	ST	—	—	—	—	—	—	—	—	—
12	B_2	—	—	0.3	0.3	—	—	0.3	ST	—	—	—	—	—	—	—	ST	—
13	B_2	—	—	—	—	—	—	ST	ST	—	—	—	—	—	—	—	—	—
14	B_2	2.0	1.7	2.0	60.0	5.0	0.6	ST	—	—	—	—	—	—	—	—	—	—
15	B_2	0.05	0.3	—	0.4	0.1	0.3	ST	—	—	—	—	—	—	—	—	—	—
		Luo with sickle-cell trait																
1	M_1 B_2	—	—	—	—	—	—	—	—	—	—	—	—	—	—	—	—	ST
2	M_1 B_2	—	—	—	—	—	—	—	—	—	—	—	—	—	—	—	—	ST
3	M_1 B_1	—	—	—	—	—	—	—	—	—	—	—	—	—	—	—	—	ST
4	M_1 B_1	—	—	—	—	—	—	—	—	—	—	—	—	—	—	—	—	ST
5	M_1 B_1	—	—	—	—	—	—	—	—	—	—	—	—	—	—	—	—	ST
6	M_1 B_1	—	—	—	—	—	—	—	—	—	—	—	—	—	—	—	—	ST
7	M_1 B_1	—	—	—	—	—	—	—	—	—	—	—	—	—	—	—	—	ST
8	M_1 B_1	0.7	—	—	—	—	—	—	—	—	—	—	—	—	—	5.0	0.5	ST
9	M_1 B_1	—	—	—	—	—	—	—	—	—	—	—	—	—	—	5.0	—	ST
10	M_1 B_1	—	—	—	—	—	—	—	—	—	—	0.03	0.1	0.03	0.03	—	—	ST
11	B_2 M_2	—	—	—	—	—	—	—	—	—	—	—	—	—	—	—	—	ST
12	B_2 M_2	—	—	—	—	—	—	—	—	—	—	—	—	—	—	—	—	ST
13	B_2 M_2	—	—	—	—	—	—	—	—	—	—	—	—	—	—	—	—	ST
14	B_2 M_2	—	—	—	—	—	—	—	—	—	—	—	—	—	—	—	—	ST
15	B_2 M_2	—	—	—	—	—	—	—	—	—	—	—	—	—	—	—	—	ST

Figures represent parasite counts in hundreds per mm.^{3} of blood.
ST = Stopped by chemotherapy.

often independent of ethnic and linguistic grouping: thus, the incidence of the sickle-cell trait among Bantu-speaking tribes ranges from 0 (among the Kamba, Chagga, etc.) to 40% (among the Amba, Simbiti, etc.). The world distribution of the sickle-cell trait is also in accordance with the view presented here that malarial endemicity is a very important factor in determining the frequency of the sickle-cell trait. The genetical and anthropological implications of this view are evident.

The fact that sickle cells should be less easily parasitized by plasmodia than are normal erythrocytes is presumably attributable to their haemoglobin component, although there may be other differences, not yet observed, between the two cell-types. Sickle-cell haemoglobin is unlike normal adult haemoglobin in important physico-chemical properties, notably in the relative insolubility of the sickle-cell haemoglobin when reduced (Perutz and Mitchison, 1950). The malaria parasite is able to metabolize haemoglobin very completely in the intact red cell, the haematin pigment remaining as a by-product of haemoglobin breakdown (Fairley and Bromfield, 1934; Moulder and Evans, 1946). That plasmodia are greatly affected by relatively small differences in their environment is suggested by their remarkable species specificity. Thus the difficulty of establishing an infection in monkeys with human malaria parasites, and vice versa, is generally recognized.

How far species differences in the haemoglobins themselves, known from immunological and other studies, are responsible for the species specificity of plasmodia it is impossible to say. However, the physico-chemical differences between human adult haemoglobin and monkey haemoglobin appear to be less pronounced than the differences between either type and sickle-cell haemoglobin. It is clear that the natural resistance to malaria among individuals with the sickle-cell trait is relative, not absolute. This is perhaps attributable to differences in the expressivity of the sickle-cell gene, which may be responsible for the production of from nearly 50% to only a very small amount of sickle-cell haemoglobin (Wells and Itano, 1951; Singer and Fisher, 1953). Moreover, the sickle-cell haemoglobin may not be evenly distributed in the cell population: most observers recognize that there are cases in which only some of the red cells are sickled even after prolonged reduction. However, even a relative resistance to malaria may be enough to help those with the sickle-cell trait through the dangerous years of early childhood, during which an active immunity to the disease is developed.

The above observations focus attention upon the importance of haemoglobin to plasmodia in the erythrocytic phase. Hence, it is worth considering whether erythrocytes containing other specialized or abnormal types of haemoglobin might be resistant to malaria also. Thus, human foetal haemoglobin differs from human adult haemoglobin in many properties. Red cells containing foetal haemoglobin continue to circulate in the newborn for the first three months of life, after which they are quite rapidly replaced by cells containing normal adult haemoglobin. It has long been known that the newborn has a considerable degree of resistance to malarial infection: Garnham (1949), for instance, found that in the Kavirondo district of Kenya at the end of the second month of life only 10% of babies were infected; after this age the percentage affected rises rapidly, until by the ninth month practically all children have the disease. The correspondence between the appearance

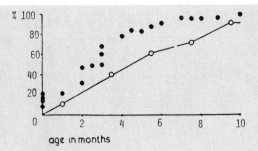

Fig. The apparent relationship between the appearance of adult-type haemoglobin (dots) and malarial infection (circles) in the newborn. Each dot represents a test on a single individual, using an alkali denaturation technique (Allison, unpublished observations); the circles represent the percentage of Luo children showing malaria parasites (Garnham, 1949).

of cells containing normal adult-type haemoglobin and malarial suscepti-bility is illustrated in the Chart. The correspondence may of course be fortuitous, but it is striking enough to merit further investigation, even though other factors, such as a milk diet deficient in *p*-aminobenzoic acid (Maegraith *et al.*, 1952; Hawking, 1953) and immunity acquired from the mother (Hackett, 1941) may play a part in the natural resistance of the newborn to malaria.

Finally, it is possible that the explanation offered above for the main-tenance of the sickle-cell trait may also apply to thalassaemia. The prob-lems presented by the two diseases are very similar; many homozygotes, and possibly some heterozygotes, are known to die of thalassaemia, and yet the condition remains remarkably common in Italy and Greece, where as many as 10% of the individuals in certain areas are affected (Bianco *et al.*, 1952). Greek and Italian authors have commented that cases of thalassaemia usually come from districts severely afflicted with malaria (Choremis *et al.*, 1951). Perhaps those who are heterozygous for the thalassaemia gene suffer less from malaria than their compatriots: the fertility of the heterozygotes appears to be greater (Bianco *et al.*, 1952). Selective advantage of the heterozygote with the sickle-cell gene, and possibly the heterozygote with the thalassaemia gene also, would explain why such high gene frequencies can be attained in the case of these conditions while other genetically transmitted abnormalities of the blood cells remain uncommon, not very much above the estimated mutation rate—for example, hereditary spherocytosis (Race, 1942).

SUMMARY

A study has been made of the relationship between the sickle-cell trait and subtertian malarial infection. It has been found that in indig-enous East Africans the sickle-cell trait affords a considerable degree of protection against subtertian malaria. The incidence of parasitaemia in 43 Ganda children with the sickle-cell trait was significantly lower than in a comparable group of 247 children without the trait. An infection with *P. falciparum* was established in 14 out of 15 Africans without the sickle-cell trait, whereas in a comparable group of 15 Africans with the trait only 2 developed parasites.

It is concluded that the abnormal erythrocytes of individuals with the sickle-cell trait are less easily parasitized by *P. falciparum* than are normal erythrocytes. Hence those who are heterozygous for the sickle-cell gene will have a selective advantage in regions where malaria is hyperendemic. This fact may explain why the sickle-cell gene remains common in these areas in spite of the elimination of genes in patients dying of sickle-cell anaemia. The implications of these observations in other branches of haematology are discussed.

REFERENCES
1. A. C. Allison. July 1954. Transactions of the Royal Society of Tropical Medical Hygiene, 48: 312-318.
2. E. A. Beet. 1946. E. Afr. Med. J. 23: 75.
3. E. A. Beat. 1947. E. Afr. Med. J. 24: 212.
4. I. Bianco, G. Montalenti, E. Silvestroni and M. Siniscalco. 1952. Ann. Eugen., Lond. 16: 299.
5. P. Brain. 1952a. Brit. Med. J. 2: 880.
6. P. Brain. 1952b. E. Afr. Med. J. 26: 925.
7. C. Choremis, N. Zervos, V. Constantinides and Leda Zannos. 1951. Lancet. 1: 1147.
8. C. Choremis, Elizabeth W. Ikin, H. Lehmann, A. E. Mourant and Leda Zannos. 1953. Lancet. 2: 909.
9. G. A. Daland and W. B. Castle. 1948. J. Lab. Clin. Med. 33: 1082.
10. G. M. Edington, 1953. Brit. Med. J. 2: 957.
11. Sir N. H. Fairley and R. J. Bromfield. 1934. Trans. Roy. Soc. Trop. Med. Hyg. 28: 141.
12. H. Foy, A. Kondi and W. Brass. 1951. E. Afr. Med. J. 28: 1.
13. P. C. C. Garnham. 1949. Ann. Trop. Med. Parasit. 43: 47.
14. L. W. Hackett. 1941. Publ. Amer. Ass. Advance. Sci. 15: 148.
15. J. B. S. Haldane. 1947. Ann. Eugen., Lond. 13: 262.
16. F. Hawking. 1953. Brit. Med. J. 1: 1201.
17. A. B. Henderson and H. E. Thornell. 1946. J. Lab. Clin. Med. 31: 769.
18. J. Humphreys. 1952. J. Trop. Med. Hyg. 55: 166.
19. J. Lambotte-Legrand and C. Lambotte-Legrand. 1951. Institut Royal Colonial Belge. Sect. d. Sci. Nat. et Med. Memoires. XIX(7) 98.
20. H. Lehmann and Marie Cutbush. 1952. Brit. Med. J. 1: 404.
21. H. Lehmann and A. H. Milne, 1949. E. Afr. Med. J. 26: 247.
22. H. Lehmann and A. B. Raper. 1949. Nature, Lond. 164: 494.
23. B. G. Maegraith, T. Deegan and E. S. Jones. 1952. Brit. Med. J. 2: 1382.
24. J. W. Moulder and E. A. Evans. 1946. J. Biol. Chem. 164: 145.
25. J. V. Neel. 1950. Cold Springs Harbor Symp. Quant. Biol. 15: 141.
26. J. V. Neel. 1952. Blood. 7: 467.
27. L. Pauling, H. A. Itano, S. J. Singer and I. C. Wells. 1949. Science. 110: 543.
28. M. F. Perutz and J. M. Mitchison. 1950. Nature, Lond. 166: 677.
29. R. R. Race. 1942. Ann. Eugen., Lond. 11: 365.

30. K. Singer and B. Fisher. 1953. Blood. 8: 270.
31. A. T. G. Thomas, G. I. Robertson and D. G. Davey. Trans. Roy. Soc. Trop. Med. Hyg. 47: 388.
32. J. M. Vandepitte and L. A. Louis. 1953. Lancet. 2: 806.
33. I. C. Wells and H. A. Itano. 1951. J. Biol. Chem. 188: 65.

(From Brit. Med. J. *1:290, 1954.)*

FURTHER READINGS

Cavalli-Sforza, L. L., and Bodmer, W. F. *The Genetics of Human Population.* San Francisco: Freeman, 1971.

Dobzhansky, T. *Genetics of the Evolutionary Process.* New York: Columbia University Press, 1971.

Harrison, G. A., Weiner, J. S., Tanner, J. M., and Barnicot, N. A. *Human Biology.* Oxford: Clarendon Press, 1964.

Lerner, I. M. *Heredity, Evolution, and Society.* San Francisco: Freeman, 1968.

Livingstone, F. B. *Abnormal Hemoglobins in Human Populations.* Chicago: Aldine-Atherton, 1967.

Salzano, F. M., and Freire-Maia, N. *Problems in Human Biology: A Study of Brazilian Populations.* Detroit: Wayne State University Press, 1970.

Stern, C. *Principles of Human Genetics.* San Francisco: Freeman, 1960.

Wallace, B. *Genetic Load, Its Biological and Conceptual Aspects.* Englewood Cliffs, N.J.: Prentice-Hall, 1970.

Appendixes

Medical History Questionnaire*

*Prepared by the Harvard Community Health Plan and the Laboratory of Computer Science, Massachusetts General Hospital

INSTRUCTIONS:
Please complete this form and forward it to us in the enclosed self-addressed envelope. This will greatly assist the Health Center in establishing your Medical Record.
This is regarded as a confidential, privileged communication. Therefore, please be frank with your answers.
Do not make any additional comments in the question and answer section of this booklet; you will have the opportunity to make additional comments in a special section at the end of the booklet.

PLEASE ANSWER EVERY QUESTION EXCEPT THOSE WITH SPECIFIC INSTRUCTIONS TO THE CONTRARY.

HOSPITALIZATIONS:
If you have been a patient in a hospital overnight or longer, please fill in below for any illness, operations or accidents.

Year	Reason

MEDICATIONS:
What medicines or drugs are you taking at present? _____
_____

Are you allergic or have you had a bad reaction to any of the following drugs:
Penicillin .... (H101) YES____ NO____
Sulfa drugs .... (H102) YES____ NO____
Phenobarbital or barbiturates .... (H103) YES____ NO____
Codeine, morphine, or demerol ...... (H104) YES____ NO____
Aspirin, empirin, or bufferin .... (H105) YES____ NO____

FAMILY HISTORY
If any blood relatives have ever had any of the conditions listed below, please check who: (If grandparents, uncles or aunts, check only whether it was on your mother's side of the family or father's side, or both sides.)

	Father	Mother	Father's side	Mother's side	Brother(s)	Sister(s)	Son(s)	Daughter(s)
	a	b	c	d	e	f	g	h
HEART ATTACK OR ANGINA (A001)								
STROKE (A002)								
HIGH BLOOD PRESSURE (A003)								
ASTHMA, HAYFEVER, HIVES, OR ECZEMA (A004)								
DIABETES (SUGAR DISEASE) (A005)								
SUICIDE OR OTHER NERVOUS DISORDER (A006)								
LIVER DISEASE (JAUNDICE) (A007)								
ANEMIA OR BLEEDING DISEASE (A008)								
KIDNEY DISEASE (A009)								
CANCER (A010)								

IS THERE SOME OTHER DISEASE OR CONDITION THAT RUNS IN YOUR FAMILY? .... (A011) YES____ NO____

IF EITHER OR BOTH OF YOUR PARENTS HAVE DIED, PLEASE CHECK THE AGE AT WHICH THEY DIED:

	Under Age 50 (a)	50-59 years (b)	60-69 years (c)	70-79 years (d)	80+ years (e)	
FATHER DIED:	___	___	___	___	___	(A012)
MOTHER DIED:	___	___	___	___	___	
	(f)	(g)	(h)	(i)	(j)	

HAVE YOU EVER HAD A TETANUS INJECTIONS? .... YES____ NO____ (A013)
A. IF YES, IN WHAT YEAR WAS IT? (A014)

1. DO YOU SMOKE CIGARETTES NOW OR HAVE YOU SMOKED CIGARETTES IN THE LAST 5 YEARS? .... (B001) YES____ NO____
   IF NO, SKIP TO QUESTION 2
   A. HOW MANY YEARS HAVE YOU SMOKED?
   Less than 5 years? ...... (B002) YES____ NO____
   5 to 10 years? .... (B003) YES____ NO____
   More than 10 years? .... (B004) YES____ NO____
   B. HOW MUCH DO YOU SMOKE?
   Nothing at the present time (B005) YES____ NO____
   Less than 1 pack a day .. (B006) YES____ NO____
   1 to 2 packs a day ..... (B008) YES____ NO____
   More than 2 packs a day? . (B009) YES____ NO____
2. WITHIN THE PAST YEAR, HAVE YOU HAD, BECAUSE OF TOO MUCH DRINKING, ANY DIFFICULTIES SUCH AS HEALTH PROBLEMS, TIME LOST FROM WORK, OR FAMILY ARGUMENTS? (B010) YES____ NO____
3. HAVE YOU GAINED 20 POUNDS SINCE AGE 20? .... (B011) YES____ NO____
4. HAVE YOU LOST MORE THAN 10 POUNDS WITHIN THE LAST 6 MONTHS? (B012) YES____ NO____
5. ARE YOU ON A SPECIAL DIET? ...... (B013) YES____ NO____
6. ARE YOU ON A WEIGHT REDUCING DIET? .... (B014) YES____ NO____
7. IN THE PAST SIX MONTHS HAVE YOU EXPERIENCED:
   Loss by separation or death, of a spouse, close relative, friend, or other important person in your life .... (B015) YES____ NO____
   Marked decline in your job, economic or physical health status .... (B016) YES____ NO____
   Change in your housing arrangement, including moves, additions or subtractions from your family .... (B017) YES____ NO____
8. DO YOU HAVE SOME SIGNIFICANT PROBLEM OR CONFLICT AT HOME, WITH YOUR FAMILY OR RELATIVES? (B018) YES____ NO____
9. HAS A DOCTOR EVER TOLD YOU THAT YOU HAVE GLAUCOMA? .... (B019) YES____ NO____
10. INDICATE WHETHER OR NOT YOU HAVE HAD ANY OF THE FOLLOWING DURING THE PAST YEAR:
    Double vision .... (B020) YES____ NO____
    Blurring eyesight which lasted more than a few minutes (B021) YES____ NO____
    Pain in either or both of your eyes .... (B022) YES____ NO____
    Temporary or permanent blindness in either eye .... (B023) YES____ NO____
    Haloes around lights .... (B024) YES____ NO____
11. ARE YOUR TEETH (OR DENTURES) CAUSING YOU SIGNIFICANT TROUBLE, OR ARE THEY IN POOR CONDITION? (B025) YES____ NO____
12. DO YOU HAVE DIFFICULTY WITH HEARING? .... (B026) YES____ NO____
13. HAS YOUR VOICE CHANGED (become rough, scratchy or hoarse) DURING THE PAST YEAR, OTHER THAN WHEN YOU HAD A COLD OR MINOR THROAT INFECTION? .... (B027) YES____ NO____
14. DO YOU USUALLY HAVE A COUGH? .... (B029) YES____ NO____
15. DO YOU BRING UP ANY MATERIAL (such as sputum, phlegm or mucus) FROM YOUR CHEST? .... (B030) YES____ NO____
16. HAVE YOU EVER COUGHED UP BLOOD? (B031) YES____ NO____
17. DO YOU GET SHORTNESS OF BREATH SUCH THAT IT **REQUIRES YOU TO STOP TO REST:**

When you are walking on level ground? .... (B032) YES____ NO____
When you are climbing a flight of stairs? .... (B033) YES____ NO____
When you are shoveling snow, or changing the sheets on a bed? ...... (B034) YES____ NO____

18. DO YOU GET SHORTNESS OF BREATH:
Which causes you to wake from sleeping? .... (B035) YES____ NO____
When you are lying quietly? (B036)YES____ NO____

19. HAVE YOU HAD WHEEZING OR WHISTLING IN YOUR CHEST IN THE PAST 2 YEARS? .... (B037) YES____ NO____
IF NO, SKIP TO QUESTION 20
A. DID THE WHEEZING START LESS THAN 3 MONTHS AGO? .... (B038) YES____ NO____
B. DO YOU STILL GET PERIODS OF WHEEZING? .... (B039) YES____ NO____

20. HAVE YOU HAD ANY OF THE FOLLOWING CONDITIONS IN THE LAST 5 YEARS?
Frequent night sweats that drench your bed clothes? .. (B040) YES____ NO____
Hay fever or frequent sneezing spells? .... (B041) YES____ NO____
Pneumonia? .... (B042) YES____ NO____
Frequent Bronchitis? ...... (B043) YES____ NO____
Pleurisy? .... (B044) YES____ NO____
Bronchial asthma? .... (B045) YES____ NO____
Emphysema? .... (B046) YES____ NO____

21. HAVE YOU HAD ANY OF THE FOLLOWING:
Tuberculosis? .... (B047) YES____ NO____
Close contact with people who have had tuberculosis (including anyone in your family) .... (B048) YES____ NO____
A positive tuberculosis skin test? .... (B049) YES____ NO____

22. HAVE YOU HAD A CHEST X-RAY WITHIN THE LAST 5 YEARS THAT WAS REPORTED AS BEING ABNORMAL? ...... (B050) YES____ NO____

23. DO YOU GET PAIN, DISCOMFORT, TIGHTNESS OR PRESSURE IN YOUR CHEST? .... (B051) YES____ NO____
IF NO, SKIP TO QUESTION 24
A. HOW OFTEN DOES IT OCCUR:
Once a month? .... (B052) YES____ NO____
Every two or three weeks? (B053) YES____ NO____
More than once a week? .. (B054) YES____ NO____
Every day? .... (B055) YES____ NO____
B. IS THE CHEST PAIN OR DISCOMFORT LOCATED:
In the middle of your chest, under the breastbone? .... (B056) YES____ NO____
On the left side only? .... (B057) YES____ NO____
On the right side only? .... (B058) YES____ NO____
On both sides? .... (B059) YES____ NO____
C. IS THE PAIN OR DISCOMFORT MADE WORSE BY BREATHING DEEPLY? .... (B060) YES____ NO____
D. DOES THIS PAIN OR DISCOMFORT COME ON AFTER YOU:
Eat a large meal? .... (B061) YES____ NO____
Become angry or excited? .. (B062) YES____ NO____
Do strenuous work or walk rapidly? .... (B063) YES____ NO____
Turn from side-to-side, lean forward or lie down? .... (B064) YES____ NO____
E. IS THE PAIN OR DISCOMFORT MADE WORSE BY SWALLOWING? (B065) YES____ NO____
F. IS THE PAIN OR DISCOMFORT RELIEVED BY RESTING? ...... (B066) YES____ NO____
G. WHEN YOU REST, DOES THE PAIN OR DISCOMFORT GO AWAY:
Immediately? .... (B067) YES____ NO____
In less than 5 minutes? .. (B068) YES____ NO____
In 5 to 30 minutes? ...... (B069) YES____ NO____
In more than 30 minutes? (B070) YES____ NO____
H. DO YOU NEED TO TAKE A MEDICINE SUCH AS NITROGLYCERIN TO RELIEVE THE PAIN? .... (B071) YES____ NO____

I. IS THE CHEST PAIN USUALLY SO PAINFUL THAT YOU ARE IN GREAT DISTRESS? .... (B072) YES____ NO____

24. DO YOU GET POUNDING, SKIPPING, THUMPING OR RACING OF YOUR HEART (palpitations and/or fluttering) WHILE YOU ARE AT REST? .... (B073) YES____ NO____

25. DO YOU FIND IT NECESSARY TO SLEEP PROPPED UP (with extra pillows or in a chair) TO HELP YOU BREATHE EASILY? (B074) YES____ NO____
IF NO, SKIP TO QUESTION 26
A. FOR HOW LONG HAVE YOU SLEPT PROPPED UP:
For less than a month? ... (B075) YES____ NO____
For a few months? .... (B076) YES____ NO____
For about a year? .... (B077) YES____ NO____
For more than a year? .... (B078) YES____ NO____

26. DO YOU GET SWELLING OF YOUR FEET OR ANKLES (which does not disappear overnight)? .... (B079) YES____ NO____

27. DO YOU CONSISTENTLY GET PAINS IN YOUR CALVES OR LOWER LEGS WHEN YOU WALK ANY DISTANCE? .... (B080) YES____ NO____
IF NO, SKIP TO QUESTION 28
A. DO THESE PAINS MAKE YOU STOP WALKING? .... (B081) YES____ NO____
B. DO THESE PAINS GO AWAY AFTER A SHORT REST (5 to 10 minutes)? .... (B082) YES____ NO____

28. DO YOU HAVE BULGING OR VISIBLE VEINS (Varicose veins) IN YOUR LEGS? (B083) YES____ NO____

29. ARE YOUR FINGERS EXCESSIVELY SENSITIVE TO COLD SO THAT THEY BECOME VERY PAINFUL, COMPLETELY WHITE, OR DARK BLUE WHEN THEY GET ONLY SLIGHTLY COLD? .... (B084) YES____ NO____

30. HAVE YOU EVER HAD SKIN ULCERS ON YOUR ANKLES WHICH TOOK MANY MONTHS TO HEAL? .... (B085) YES____ NO____

31. HAVE YOU EVER TAKEN MEDICINE:
For your heart? .... (B086) YES____ NO____
For high blood pressure? .. (B087) YES____ NO____
To help thin your blood? .. (B088) YES____ NO____
For the purpose of losing water? .... (B089) YES____ NO____

32. HAS A DOCTOR EVER TOLD YOU THAT YOU HAD:
Heart murmur? .... (B090) YES____ NO____
Enlarged heart? .... (B091) YES____ NO____
High blood pressure? ..... (B092) YES____ NO____
A heart attack? .... (B093) YES____ NO____
Rheumatic fever? .... (B094) YES____ NO____
Angina or angina pectoris? (B095) YES____ NO____
Phlebitis, thrombophlebitis or "milk leg"? .... (B096) YES____ NO____
Trouble with your circulation (B097) YES____ NO____

33. IN THE LAST YEAR, HAVE YOU HAD:
A persistent sore tongue? (B098) YES____ NO____
Bleeding gums that have been very troublesome? (B099) YES____ NO____
A choking feeling or a lump in the throat when not eating? .... (B100) YES____ NO____
Trouble swallowing food or liquids? .... (B101) YES____ NO____
Food or liquid stick in your throat while swallowing? (B102) YES____ NO____

34. DO YOU GET AN UPSET STOMACH, PAINS IN YOUR STOMACH OR ABDOMINAL DISTRESS MORE THAN ONCE A A WEEK? .... (C005) YES____ NO____
IF NO, SKIP TO QUESTION 36
A. DO THE PAINS OCCUR:
Every day? .... (C006) YES____ NO____
Every few days? .... (C007) YES____ NO____
Every week or two? ...... (C008) YES____ NO____
Occasionally? .... (C009) YES____ NO____
Only during your menstrual periods? .... (C010) YES____ NO____
B. ARE THESE PAINS LOCATED:
Above the navel? .... (C011) YES____ NO____
Below the navel? .... (C012) YES____ NO____
On the right side? .... (C013) YES____ NO____
On the left side? .... (C014) YES____ NO____
Throughout the stomach? .. (C015) YES____ NO____

C. DO THESE PAINS IN YOUR STOM-
ACH OR ABDOMEN FEEL:
Dull? .... (C016) YES____ NO____
Sharp? .... (C017) YES____ NO____
Crampy? .... (C018) YES____ NO____
Other kind of feeling? .... (C019) YES____ NO____
D. DO THESE PAINS COME ON:
At the time of, or directly
after, eating a meal? ..... (C020) YES____ NO____
One or two hours after eat-
ing? .... (C021) YES____ NO____
At no particular time? .... (C022) YES____ NO____
E. DO THESE STOMACH PAINS:
Become worse on bending or
lying down? .... (C023) YES____ NO____
Keep you from going to
sleep? .... (C024) YES____ NO____
Awaken you from sleep? .. (C025) YES____ NO____
Come on after eating fried
or fatty foods? .... (C026) YES____ NO____
F. ARE THESE PAINS RELIEVED BY:
Taking milk, soda, Tums
or Maalox (antacids)? .... (C027) YES____ NO____
Eating? .... (C028) YES____ NO____
A bowel movement? ...... (C029) YES____ NO____
36. DO YOU HAVE ATTACKS OF NAUSEA OR
VOMITING MORE THAN ONCE A
MONTH? .... (C030) YES____ NO____
37. HAVE YOU EVER VOMITED BLOOD OR
MATERIAL THAT LOOKS LIKE COFFEE
GROUNDS? .... (C035) YES____ NO____
38. HAVE YOUR SKIN OR EYES EVER BEEN
YELLOW OR HAVE YOU BEEN TOLD BY A
DOCTOR THAT YOU HAD JAUNDICE? .. (C036) YES____ NO____
39. DO YOU HAVE TROUBLE WITH:
Constipation? .... (C037) YES____ NO____
Diarrhea? .... (C038) YES____ NO____
Rectal pain? .... (C039) YES____ NO____
Straining on expelling a
bowel movement? .... (C040) YES____ NO____
Any other abnormality with
your bowel movement? .... (C041) YES____ NO____
40. DO YOU USE A LAXATIVE FREQUENTLY? (C042) YES____ NO____
41. HAVE YOU EVER HAD BOWEL MOVE-
MENTS THAT WERE AS BLACK AS COAL
OR TAR? .... (C043) YES____ NO____
IF NO, SKIP TO QUESTION 42
A. WERE YOU TAKING IRON OR VITA-
MINS AT THE TIME OF THE BLACK
BOWEL MOVEMENTS? .... (C044) YES____ NO____
42. HAVE YOU EVER HAD BLOOD IN YOUR
BOWEL MOVEMENTS? .... (C045) YES____ NO____
43. HAS A DOCTOR EVER TOLD YOU THAT
YOU HAD:
An ulcer (stomach or duode-
nal)? .... (C046) YES____ NO____
Gallstones or gall bladder
disease? .... (C047) YES____ NO____
Cirrhosis, hepatitis or some
other liver disease? ...... (C048) YES____ NO____
Inflamed stomach (gastritis)? (C049) YES____ NO____
Nervous stomach? .... (C050) YES____ NO____
Pancreatitis? .... (C051) YES____ NO____
Intestinal disease (bowel or
colon disease)? .... (C052) YES____ NO____
Hemorrhoids or piles? ...... (C053) YES____ NO____
Worms or parasites? ...... (C054) YES____ NO____
Dysentery or serious diar-
rhea? .... (C055) YES____ NO____
44. HAVE YOU EVER HAD AN OPERATION
ON YOUR:
Stomach? .... (C056) YES____ NO____
Gallbladder? .... (C057) YES____ NO____
Appendix? .... (C058) YES____ NO____
Colon (bowel)? .... (C059) YES____ NO____
Anus (rectum)? .... (C060) YES____ NO____
Other parts of your abdomen? (C061) YES____ NO____
45. HAVE YOU EVER HAD ANY OF THE FOL-
LOWING X-RAYS IN THE LAST 4 YEARS:
Stomach? .... (C062) YES____ NO____
Gallbladder? .... (C063) YES____ NO____
Intestines (upper gastrointes-
tinal series, barium enema)? (C064) YES____ NO____

46. HAVE YOU BROKEN MORE THAN TWO
BONES DURING YOUR LIFETIME? .... (C065) YES____ NO____
47. DO YOU GET STIFFNESS IN YOUR
JOINTS UPON AWAKENING? .... (C066) YES____ NO____
48. HAS A DOCTOR EVER TOLD YOU THAT
YOU HAD "ARTHRITIS"? .... (C067) YES____ NO____
49. DO YOU GET SEVERE BACK PAINS THAT
PREVENT YOU FROM DOING YOUR NOR-
MAL WORK? .... (C068) YES____ NO____
IF NO, SKIP TO QUESTION 50
A. HOW OFTEN DO YOU GET THESE
BACK PAINS:
Frequently (every day)? .. (C069) YES____ NO____
Occasionally (some time
each week)? .... (C070) YES____ NO____
After doing heavy work? .. (C071) YES____ NO____
Rarely? .... (C072) YES____ NO____
B. DO THESE PAINS USUALLY START
IN YOUR LOWER SPINE AND PASS
DOWN THE BACK OF EITHER OR
BOTH LEGS? .... (C073) YES____ NO____
50. HAS A DOCTOR EVER TOLD YOU THAT
YOU HAD GOUT? .... (C074) YES____ NO____
51. HAVE YOU EVER HAD AN OPERATION
ON YOUR BONES OR JOINTS? ...... (C075) YES____ NO____
52. HAVE YOU EVER HAD RED, TENDER OR
SWOLLEN JOINTS? .... (C076) YES____ NO____
53. DO YOU GET PAIN IN YOUR BONES OR
JOINTS? .... (C077) YES____ NO____
IF NO, SKIP TO QUESTION 54
A. IS THIS PAIN OFTEN SO SEVERE
THAT IT PREVENTS YOU FROM SAT-
ISFACTORILY MOVING YOUR ARM
OR LEG? .... (C078) YES____ NO____
B. DOES THIS PAIN INVOLVE MANY
JOINTS? .... (C079) YES____ NO____
C. DOES WALKING INCREASE THE
PAIN? .... (C080) YES____ NO____
D. DOES WALKING RELIEVE THE PAIN? (C081) YES____ NO____
E. DOES ASPIRIN, ANACIN, BUFFERIN
OR OTHER MILD PAIN MEDICATION
RELIEVE THE PAIN? .... (C082) YES____ NO____
54. IN THE PAST YEAR, DID YOU HAVE:
Burning or pain on urination? (C083) YES____ NO____
Difficulty in starting urina-
tion? .... (C084) YES____ NO____
Unexpected loss of urine
when you cough, sneeze,
laugh, etc? .... (C085) YES____ NO____
Blood in your urine? ...... (C086) YES____ NO____
Dark urine? .... (C087) YES____ NO____
Pus in your urine? .... (C088) YES____ NO____
55. DO YOU USUALLY GET UP AT NIGHT TO
URINATE? .... (C089) YES____ NO____
IF NO, SKIP TO QUESTION 56
A. DO YOU USUALLY GET UP MORE
THAN 2 TIMES A NIGHT? ...... (C090) YES____ NO____
B. FOR HOW LONG HAVE YOU BEEN
GETTING UP TO URINATE:
For less than 6 months? .. (C091) YES____ NO____
For about 6 months to 1
year? .... (C092) YES____ NO____
For more than 1 year? .... (C093) YES____ NO____
56. HAS A DOCTOR EVER TOLD YOU THAT
YOU HAD:
Prostate trouble? .... (C094) YES____ NO____
Kidney or bladder infection
that was very difficult to
clear up or which recurred
frequently? .... (C095) YES____ NO____
Kidney or bladder stones
(gravel)? .... (C096) YES____ NO____
Venereal disease ("VD")? .. (C097) YES____ NO____
Hernia? .... (C098) YES____ NO____
57. HAVE YOU EVER HAD A BLADDER OR A
KIDNEY OPERATION? .... (C099) YES____ NO____
58. HAVE YOU EVER HAD A KIDNEY X-RAY
(Intravenous Pyelogram)? .... (C100) YES____ NO____
59. ARE THERE TIMES WHEN YOU FEEL
THAT YOU HAVE TO URINATE BUT FIND
THAT YOU CANNOT PASS ANY URINE? (D001) YES____ NO____
60. DOES YOUR URINE OFTEN COME OUT
IN DRIBBLES, RATHER THAN IN A
STRONG STREAM? .... (D002) YES____ NO____

61. HAVE YOU EVER BEEN TOLD THAT YOU
WERE ANEMIC? .... (D003) YES___ NO___
IF NO, SKIP TO QUESTION 62
   A. HAVE YOU TAKEN ANY IRON
MEDICINE OR OTHER MEDICA-
TIONS FOR ANEMIA IN THE
PAST YEAR? .... (D004) YES___ NO___
62. DO YOU OFTEN GET MANY BLACK AND
BLUE SPOTS WITHOUT APPARENT
REASON? .... (D005) YES___ NO___
63. DO YOU BLEED FOR A VERY LONG
TIME WITHOUT STOPPING WHEN YOU
INJURE YOURSELF OR WHEN YOU HAVE
SURGERY OR TOOTH EXTRACTIONS ... (D006) YES___ NO___
64. HAVE YOU NOTICED ENLARGED GLANDS
OR LYMPH NODES DURING THE PAST
YEAR? .... (D007) YES___ NO___
IF NO, SKIP TO QUESTION 65
   A. IN WHICH OF THE FOLLOWING
PARTS OF YOUR BODY WERE
THE ENLARGED NODES:
      Neck? .... (D008) YES___ NO___
      Armpit? .... (D009) YES___ NO___
      Groin? .... (D010) YES___ NO___
      Other parts of the body? .. (D011) YES___ NO___
65. HAVE YOU EVER RECEIVED A BLOOD
TRANSFUSION? .... (D012) YES___ NO___
   A. DID YOU HAVE A RASH OR
OTHER REACTION TO THE
BLOOD? .... (D013) YES___ NO___
66. HAVE YOU HAD VITAMIN B-12 INJEC-
TIONS IN THE PAST YEAR? .... (D014) YES___ NO___
67. DO YOUR HANDS TREMBLE OR SHAKE
MOST OF THE TIME? .... (D015) YES___ NO___
68. HAVE YOU EVER HAD SUGAR IN YOUR
URINE? .... (D016) YES___ NO___
69. HAVE YOU NOTICED ANY RECENT
CHANGE IN THE COLOR OF YOUR
SKIN? .... (D017) YES___ NO___
IF NO, SKIP TO QUESTION 70
   A. HAS THE COLOR OF YOUR SKIN
BECOME:
      Darker (other than suntan)? (D018) YES___ NO___
      Lighter or more pale? .... (D019) YES___ NO___
      Yellow? .... (D020) YES___ NO___
      Other change? .... (D021) YES___ NO___
70. HAVE YOU NOTICED ANY CHANGE IN
THE TEXTURE OR FEEL OF YOUR
SKIN? .... (D022) YES___ NO___
71. HAVE YOU RECENTLY BEGUN TO DRINK
MUCH MORE WATER OR LIQUIDS THAN
YOU USED TO? .... (D023) YES___ NO___
72. HAS YOUR DOCTOR EVER TOLD YOU
THAT YOU HAVE HAD ANY OF THE
FOLLOWING:
      Diabetes (sugar disease)? . (D024) YES___ NO___
      Overactive Thyroid? ..... (D025) YES___ NO___
      Low metabolism or under-
      active thyroid? .... (D026) YES___ NO___
      Goiter (enlarged thyroid)? . (D027) YES___ NO___
      High cholesterol? .... (D028) YES___ NO___
73. HAVE YOU NOTICED ANY OF THE
FOLLOWING DURING THE LAST SIX
MONTHS:
      Extreme discomfort in hot
      weather? .... (D029) YES___ NO___
      Extreme discomfort in cold
      weather? .... (D030) YES___ NO___
74. HAVE YOU NOTICED THAT YOUR EYES
HAVE BULGED FORWARD:
      All your life? .... (D031) YES___ NO___
      Within the past few years
      only? .... (D032) YES___ NO___
75. HAVE YOU HAD ANY ANNOYING SKIN
RASHES IN THE PAST YEAR WHICH
LASTED FOR ONE MONTH OR LONGER? (D033) YES___ NO___
76. DO YOU GET FREQUENT SKIN INFEC-
TIONS OR BOILS? .... (D034) YES___ NO___
77. HAVE YOU EVER HAD HIVES, WELTS
OR SWELLING OF YOUR SKIN? .... (D035) YES___ NO___
78. IN THE PAST YEAR HAVE YOU NOTICED
ANY:
      New growths on your skin? (D036) YES___ NO___
      Moles which became larger
      or darker? .... (D037) YES___ NO___
      Sores that will not heal? .. (D038) YES___ NO___

79. ARE YOU ALLERGIC TO OR HAVE YOU
EVER DEVELOPED A RASH, ECZEMA,
WHEEZING OR NASAL BLOCKAGE FROM
ANY OF THE FOLLOWING:
      Detergents, soaps, sham-
      poos? .... (D039) YES___ NO___
      Cosmetics or hair dyes? .. (D040) YES___ NO___
      Seafoods, spices or other
      foods (causing skin
      rashes)? .... (D041) YES___ NO___
      Penicillin? .... (D042) YES___ NO___
      Some other drug or medi-
      cine? .... (D043) YES___ NO___
80. HAVE YOU EVER WORKED WHERE YOU
WERE OFTEN AROUND ANY OF THE
FOLLOWING:
      Chemicals, cleaning fluids or
      solvents? .... (D044) YES___ NO___
      Insect or plant sprays? ... (D045) YES___ NO___
      Ammonia, chlorine, ozone or
      nitrous gases? .... (D046) YES___ NO___
      Plastic or resin fumes? ... (D047) YES___ NO___
      Lead or metal fumes? .... (D048) YES___ NO___
      X-rays, radioactivity or ultra-
      violet radiation? .... (D049) YES___ NO___
      Beryllium, asbestos, poly-
      urethanes? .... (D050) YES___ NO___
81. HAVE YOU EVER HAD RADIOTHERAPY? (D051) YES___ NO___
82. DO YOU HAVE WHEEZING, A STUFFY
NOSE, RASH, HIVES, ECZEMA OR
THROAT SWELLING THAT OCCURS ONLY
AT CERTAIN SEASONS OF THE YEAR? . (D052) YES___ NO___
83. DO YOU GET VERY BAD HEADACHES
MORE THAN ONCE A WEEK? .... (D053) YES___ NO___
IF NO, SKIP TO QUESTION 84
   A. DO YOU FEEL THESE HEADACHES
HAVE BEEN GETTING WORSE IN
THE PAST SIX MONTHS? .... (D074) YES___ NO___
   B. HAVE YOU BEEN TOLD THAT YOU
HAVE MIGRAINE HEADACHES? .... (D075) YES___ NO___
   C. DO YOU RELATE THE HEADACHES
TO TENSION? .... (D076) YES___ NO___
   D. ARE THE HEADACHES RELIVED BY:
      Aspirin, Bufferin, Anacin, Ex-
      cedrin, Darvon or other mild
      headache remedies? .... (D077) YES___ NO___
84 DO YOU OFTEN HAVE DIZZY SPELLS
WHICH INTERFERE WITH YOUR WORK
IN YOUR NORMAL DAY'S ACTIVITIES? (D078) YES___ NO___
IF NO, SKIP TO QUESTION 85
   A. ARE ANY OF THE FOLLOWING AS-
SOCIATED WITH YOUR DIZZY
SPELLS:
      Lightheadedness? .... (D079) YES___ NO___
      Whirling or spinning sensa-
      tions? .... (D080) YES___ NO___
      Objects rotating or moving
      about? .... (D081) YES___ NO___
      Deafness? .... (D082) YES___ NO___
      Ringing in your ears, or
      noises? .... (D083) YES___ NO___
      Nausea or vomiting? ...... (D084) YES___ NO___
      Staggering or difficulty walk-
      ing? .... (D085) YES___ NO___
   B. IS THE DIZZINESS BROUGHT ON
BY:
      Moving your head? ...... (D086) YES___ NO___
      Changing positions, for ex-
      ample, standing up? .... (D087) YES___ NO___
   C. HOW LONG DO THE ATTACKS LAST:
      A couple of minutes or less? (D088) YES___ NO___
      An hour? .... (D089) YES___ NO___
      A couple of hours or more? (D090) YES___ NO___
   D. HAVE YOU EVER FALLEN DOWN OR
TO THE SIDE BECAUSE OF A DIZZY
SPELL? .... (D091) YES___ NO___
   E. ARE THEY MADE WORSE BY MOV-
ING YOUR HEAD? .... (D092) YES___ NO___
85. DO YOU HAVE, OR HAVE YOU HAD CON-
VULSIONS (seizures, Epilepsy, or fits)
WITHIN THE LAST 2 YEARS? .... (D093) YES___ NO___

86. DO YOU HAVE WEAKNESS, STIFFNESS OR PARALYSIS OF ANY LIMB? .... (D094) YES____ NO____
87. HAVE YOU EVER HAD A STROKE? .... (D095) YES____ NO____
88. IN THE PAST YEAR, HAVE YOU FAINTED OR PASSED OUT? .... (D096) YES____ NO____
89. ARE YOU DEPRESSED, UPHAPPY OR LACKING ENTHUSIASM MOST OF THE TIME? .... (D097) YES____ NO____
90. ARE YOU ANXIOUS, WORRIED, FEARFUL AND TENSE MOST OF THE TIME? ..... (D098) YES____ NO____
91. DO YOU FEEL THAT MANY OF YOUR COMPLAINTS ARE A RESULT OF YOUR BEING ANXIOUS OR NERVOUS? ...... (D099) YES____ NO____
92. DO YOU HAVE DIFFICULTY SLEEPING AT NIGHT? .... (D100) YES____ NO____
IF NO, SKIP TO QUESTION 93
   A. IS THIS BECAUSE YOU:
      Have trouble getting to sleep? .... (E001) YES____ NO____
      Awaken in the middle of night? .... (E002) YES____ NO____
      Awaken too early in the morning? .... (E003) YES____ NO____
93. ARE YOU CONSTANTLY TIRED AND EXHAUSTED? .... (E004) YES____ NO____
94. DOES NERVOUSNESS CAUSE YOU DIFFICULTY:
      With eating? .... (E005) YES____ NO____
      Concentrating on things? .. (E006) YES____ NO____
95. HAVE YOU NOTED A DECREASE IN YOUR APPETITE OR A WEIGHT LOSS? ...... (E007) YES____ NO____
96. DO YOU OFTEN FEEL THAT LIFE IS NOT WORTH LIVING? .... (E008) YES____ NO____
97. HAVE YOU EVER WANTED TO OR ATTEMPTED TO HARM YOURSELF? ...... (E009) YES____ NO____
98. DO YOU HAVE UPSETTING, UNUSUAL, OR BIZARRE THOUGHTS GOING ON IN YOUR MIND THAT YOU ARE UNABLE TO STOP? .... (E010) YES____ NO____
99. HAVE YOU EVER SOUGHT THE HELP OF A DOCTOR FOR A NERVOUS DISORDER OR DEPRESSION? .... (E011) YES____ NO____
IF NO, SKIP TO QUESTION 100
   A. WERE YOU HOSPITALIZED FOR THIS NERVOUS DISORDER OR DEPRESSION? .... (E012) YES____ NO____
100. ARE YOU NOW:
      A student? .... (F001) YES____ NO____
      A housewife? .... (F002) YES____ NO____
      Unemployed, temporarily? .. (F003) YES____ NO____
      Disabled, temporarily? .... (F004) YES____ NO____
      Retired? .... (F005) YES____ NO____
      Self-employed? .... (F006) YES____ NO____
      Employed? .... (F007) YES____ NO____
101. WHAT TYPE OF WORK DO YOU DO WHEN YOU ARE (or were) WORKING? (Please list your specific job, such as carpenter, plumber, high school teacher, etc., rather than your title or general line of work, such as craftsman, educator.) _____

102. CIRCLE THE NUMBER THAT CORRESPONDS TO THE HIGHEST GRADE OF SCHOOL THAT YOU COMPLETED:
1 2 3 4 5 6 7 8   9 10 11 12   1 2 3   1 2 3 4   1 2 3 4 4+
Grade School   High School   Vocational College   Graduate
                              School   (undergraduate) School
                                                        (F008)

IN CASES OF EMERGENCY, PLEASE INDICATE BELOW THE PERSON TO BE CONTACTED:

NAME _____ RELATIONSHIP _____

ADDRESS _____
         No.   Street   Apt. No.

_____
         town   State   Zip Code

TELEPHONE NUMBER _____

ARE THERE ANY ANSWERS YOU WOULD LIKE TO EXPAND UPON, OR DO YOU HAVE ANY HEALTH OR HEALTH-RELATED PROBLEMS WHICH ARE NOT INCLUDED IN THIS QUESTIONNAIRE OR WHICH YOU WOULD LIKE TO DISCUSS WITH A PLAN PHYSICIAN? ....

_____

_____

_____

_____

_____

_____

_____

_____

_____

_____

Date: _____ Signature: _____

NOTE: IF YOU ARE **FEMALE,** PLEASE GO ON TO THE NEXT SECTION. IF YOU ARE **MALE,** YOU HAVE FINISHED THE QUESTIONNAIRE. PLEASE RETURN IT TO THE HARVARD COMMUNITY HEALTH PLAN AS SOON AS POSSIBLE, USING THE ENCLOSED ENVELOPE. THANK YOU VERY MUCH FOR YOUR CO-OPERATION. THIS INFORMATION WILL BE ATTACHED TO YOUR RECORD AND IS ENTIRELY CONFIDENTIAL AND PRIVATE.

THIS SECTION TO BE COMPLETED BY FEMALE PATIENTS ONLY. PLEASE ANSWER EVERY QUESTION EXCEPT THOSE WITH SPECIFIC INSTRUCTIONS TO THE CONTRARY.
1. HAVE YOU FELT ANY LUMPS IN YOUR BREASTS IN THE PAST 2 YEARS? .... (G001) YES____ NO____
IF NO, SKIP TO QUESTION 2.
   A. ARE THE LUMPS PRESENT NOW? (G002) YES____ NO____
   B. FOR HOW LONG HAVE YOU NOTICED THE PRESENCE OF THESE LUMPS?
      Less than 6 months? (G003) YES____ NO____
      Between 6 months and 1 year? .... (G004) YES____ NO____
      More than 1 year? ..... (G005) YES____ NO____
2. HAVE YOU NOTICED ANY DISCHARGE FROM THE BREAST NIPPLES (other than when you were pregnant)? .... (G006) YES____ NO____
3. HAVE YOU HAD ANY SWELLING, PAIN, OR TENDERNESS IN YOUR BREAST OTHER THAN AROUND THE TIME OF YOUR PERIOD? .... (G007) YES____ NO____
4. HAVE YOU NOTICED AN INCREASE IN THE AMOUNT OF HAIR ON YOUR BODY DURING THE PAST 6 MONTHS? .. (G008) YES____ NO____
5. DID YOUR MENSTRUAL PERIODS START:
      Before age 12? .... (G009) YES____ NO____
      Between ages 12 and 16? (G010) YES____ NO____
      After age 16? .... (G011) YES____ NO____
6. HAVE YOU HAD IRREGULAR OR ABNORMAL MENSTRUAL PERIODS DURING ANY PART OF THE LAST YEAR? .... (G012) YES____ NO____
IF NO, SKIP TO QUESTION 7.
   A. ARE YOUR PERIODS STILL IRREGULAR? .... (G103) YES____ NO____
7. ARE YOU HAVING MUCH MORE PAIN WITH YOUR MENSTRUAL PERIODS THAN YOU USED TO? .... (G014) YES____ NO____
8. HAVE YOU STOPPED HAVING MENSTRUAL PERIODS? .... (G015) YES____ NO____
IF NO, SKIP TO QUESTION 9.
   A. AT WHAT AGE?
      Before you were 35? ...... (G016) YES____ NO____
      When you were 35 to 45? .. (G017) YES____ NO____
      When you were over 45? .. (G018) YES____ NO____

HAVE YOU NOTICED ANY BLEEDING THAT WAS NOT A PERIOD, OR ANY VAGINAL BLEEDING BETWEEN YOUR PERIODS? (G019) YES_____ NO_____

HAVE YOU AN INCREASED DISCHARGE (other than blood) FROM YOUR VAGINA? (G020) YES_____ NO_____

HAVE YOU EVER HAD AN INFECTION OF YOUR TUBES? (G021) YES_____ NO_____

ARE YOU TAKING ANY HORMONE PILLS FOR BIRTH CONTROL OR TO CONTROL "HOT FLASHES"? (G022) YES_____ NO_____

HAVE YOU TRIED TO HAVE CHILDREN BUT BEEN UNABLE TO BECOME PREG-NANT? (G023) YES_____ NO_____

HAVE YOU EVER HAD:

A hysterectomy?	(G024) YES_____	NO_____
Breast surgery?	(G025) YES_____	NO_____
Removal of an ovary only?	(G026) YES_____	NO_____
A bladder "repair" or "sus-pension" operation?	(G027) YES_____	NO_____
Cancer (not a "tumor") of your cervix or uterus?	(G028) YES_____	NO_____
X-ray or radium treatment of your female organs?	(G029) YES_____	NO_____

DID YOU EVER HAVE HIGH BLOOD PRESSURE DURING PREGNANCY? (G030) YES_____ NO_____

DID ANY OF YOUR BABIES WEIGH 9 POUNDS OR MORE AT BIRTH? (G031) YES_____ NO_____

TO YOUR KNOWLEDGE, HAVE YOU EVER HAD GERMAN MEASLES? (G032) YES_____ NO_____

THIS QUESTIONNAIRE IS NOW FINISHED. PLEASE BE CERTAIN THAT YOU RETURN IT TO THE HARVARD COMMUNITY HEALTH PLAN AS SOON AS POSSIBLE, USING THE SPECIAL MAILING ENVELOPE. THANK YOU - YOUR COOPERATION IS VERY MUCH APPRECIATED. THIS COMPLETED QUESTIONNAIRE WILL BE ATTACHED TO YOUR MEDICAL RECORD AND IS ENTIRELY CONFIDENTIAL AND PRIVATE.

II   Electrophoresis

Many biochemical compounds can be dissociated into ions. These include large molecules like proteins, that have many positive and negative charges. When placed in an electric field, these molecules will migrate according to their net charge. The technique called *electrophoresis* was introduced by Tiselius in 1937 to separate, identify, and characterize proteins and other macromolecules.

FREE ELECTROPHORESIS

The Tiselius apparatus for free electrophoresis uses a U-shaped cell with electrodes inserted at each end (Fig. II-1). When the field is produced, the mixture of proteins begins to migrate, and the movement of the various components can be followed by the changes in the refractive index or by ultraviolet absorption throughout the length of the cell.

Proteins will migrate to one of the two poles according to the sign of their net charge, with a speed that depends on the value of the charge and the strength of the electric field (in volts per distance in centimeters between electrodes). This migration will be opposed by the friction of the molecules against the medium, a friction which varies with the viscosity of the medium and the cross-sectional width of the migrating molecule. Because different proteins have different charges and sizes, they will separate in the electric field.

As dissociation is reversible (Fig. II-2), the net charge will depend on the pH of the solution. For each protein a pH can be found such that the protein has no net charge (the *isoelectric* point) and thus will not migrate.

The buffer solution has another effect on the electrophoretic mobility. Charged particles are not truly distributed at random, as each positive charge

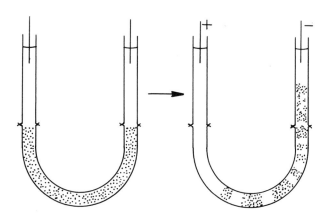

Fig. II-1. Tiselius-type cell for free electophoresis.

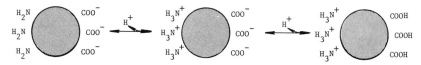

Fig. II-2. Dissociation of proteins.

attracts a cloud of negative charges and each negative charge attracts a cloud of positive charges. The charges interact and oppose migration. Therefore, when the electrophoretic mobility of a protein is defined, it is important to specify the conditions used for the measurement, such as pH, temperature, and composition of the medium. When different media are compared, the concentration of the solutions must be expressed as to include this charge interaction. This is done by using the ionic strength, $r/2$, which is half the sum of the concentration of each ion, multiplied by the square of its charge.

$$r/2 = 1/2 \; \Sigma \; C_i z_i^2$$

where C is the concentration and z is the charge.

A full theoretical treatment of the electrophoretic migration of large molecules in solution has been made, and electrophoresis has been used for some basic investigations into the shape of protein molecules. There are a number of complications such as diffusion, convection currents, and the migration of water dragged by the migration of small ions (electroosmosis), so that a full theoretical analysis loses importance. Still, free electrophoresis can be used to check the homogeneity of a protein preparation. If the preparation is a mixture, it may separate. If the field is reversed, the band containing protein may be further sharpened if the protein is pure or spread out if it contains more than one component with very similar migration rates. By disconnecting the field, the diffusion of protein molecules can be measured, providing important information with relation to size and shape.

About the same time as Tiselius was developing free electrophoresis in Sweden, Koning in Brazil invented paper electrophoresis (Fig. II-3). A strip of paper, moistened in buffer, is placed between two chambers containing buffer and electrodes. The sample is applied to the filter paper as a streak. When the current is connected, the different components will migrate at different rates. Suitable stains can be used to detect the components, and the intensity of the lines can be measured with a photoelectric densitometer to calculate concentrations.

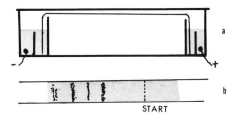

Fig. II-3. (a) Paper electrophoresis apparatus and (b) the paper strip after staining.

The filter paper acts as a solid support for the buffer, thus avoiding convection currents and making the whole apparatus quite simple to set up. It also interacts with the migrating molecules, not just by offering mechanical resistance but also by adsorption of the ions on the surface of the cellulose molecules such that adsorption varies for different components. Paper has been replaced recently by other supports which interact with the migrating molecules and result in better separation. Cellulose-acetate, agar, and partially hydrolyzed starch have all been used.

A major development was introduced in 1964 by Orenstein and Davis: acrylamide gel or *disc electrophoresis.* Acrylamide solutions of different concentrations can polymerize to give gels with pores ranging from 1.2 to 4.4 mm. These pores may be filled with electrolyte solvent. Generally this is done in a narrow glass tube, producing a clear cylinder of the gel. A sample is added to one end, and the tube is connected through two electrolyte chambers to a direct current power supply (Fig. II-4). The components migrate in this gel as very sharp bands. This process separates, in a better manner, many more components than other forms of electrophoresis. It is now a standard method of checking the homogeneity of proteins.

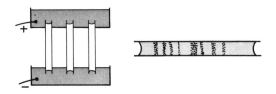

Fig. II-4. (a) Disc electrophoresis apparatus and (b) the gel after staining.

The bands can be stained to appear as sharp discs, which gives the name to the process. The discs may be cut out, eluted, and assayed (for enzymatic activity or radioactivity).

A very important application of acrylamine electrophoresis is the determination of molecular weights of macromolecules. The mobility of proteins (in sodium docecyl sulfate solution) and nucleic acids was found to be proportional to the log of their molecular weights. Molecular weights can be estimated by comparison with known standards.

BIBLIOGRAPHY

Block, R. J., Durrum, E. L., and Zweigh, G. *A Manual of Paper Chromatograph and Paper Electrophoresis* (2nd ed.). New York: Academic, 1958.

Maurer, H. R. *Disc Electrophoresis* (2nd ed.). Berlin: de Gruyter, 1971.

Shaw, D. J. *Electrophoresis.* New York: Academic, 1969.

Sirbasky, D. A., and Buchanan, J. M. Patterns of ribonucleic acid synthesis in T5 infected Escherichia coli II of high molecular weight ribonucleic acid species by disc electrophoresis on acrylamide gel columns. *J. Biol. Chem.* 245:2679, 1970.

Smith, I. *Chromatographic and Electrophoretic Techniques.* New York: Interscience, 1960.

Van Holde, K. E. *Physical Biochemistry.* Englewood Cliffs, N.J.: Prentice-Hall, 1971.

Weber, K., and Osborn, M. The reliability of molecular weight determination by dodecyl sulfate-polyacrylamide gel electrophoresis. *J. Biol. Chem.* 244:4406, 1969.

III   Centrifugation

THEORETICAL ASPECTS

The basic idea behind centrifugation is that particles suspended in a medium may be separated if subject to a centrifugal force. This is generally accomplished by putting the solution in a container at the edge of a rotor which turns at set speeds. Sedimentation occurs as the particles move at a certain velocity or *sedimentation rate* through the medium, which rate depends on the force G in such a way that

$$G = \omega^2 r = 4 \pi^2 \, (\text{rpm})^2 \, r/3600$$

where ω = angular velocity in radians per second, r = distance of particles from axis of rotation, and rpm = revolutions per minute of the rotor. Dividing G by the gravitational force, g, yields the relative centrifugal force (RCF), a measure of the intensity of the centrifugal force. An easy way to calculate RCF is given in Figure III-1. When the particles have all come to a rest at the bottom of the container, they form the *pellet*, with a supernatant solution lying above.

The sedimentation rate is affected by various factors such as particle shape, size (determined by the radius), relative density, and medium viscosity. The effect of these factors on sedimentation velocity (s) is given by

$$s = (2r_p)^2 \, (p' - p)/18 \, N \, (f/f_0)$$

where r_p = average particle radius, p' = particle density, p = medium density, N = medium viscosity, and f/f_0 = friction factor (sedimentation velocity of a hypothetical spherical particle/velocity of actual particles). The sedimentation coefficient used for sedimentation rate description is determined at a standard temperature in water of 20°C and is denoted as $s_{20,w}$.

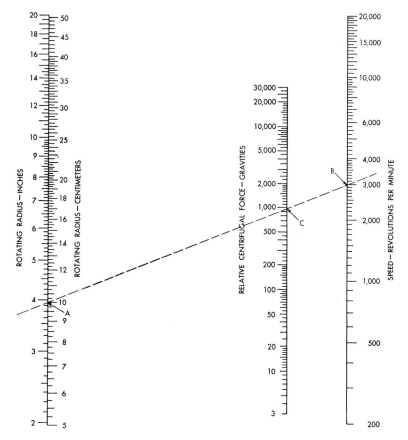

Fig. III-1. Nomogram for computing centrifugal force.

Centrifuges, then, can be used to separate particles from the suspending medium. Using much higher g's, it is possible to separate or detect macromolecular components in a mixture. From the measurement of sedimentation coefficients, molecular weights can be calculated.

DETERMINATION OF MOLECULAR WEIGHT

There are basically two ways to determine molecular weight. First, if the sedimentation coefficient (s) can be determined by sedimentation velocity as described above, one uses the Svedberg equation:

$$M = RTs/D\,(1-vp)$$

where R = gas constant, T = absolute temperature, D = diffusion constant of solute, and 1 – vp is a buoyancy term in which v = partial specific volume of solute and p = density of solvent.

The second way of finding molecular weight is called *sedimentation equilibrium*. This involves spinning at low speeds to allow the force of sedimentation to equal that of diffusion. In this case

$$M = 2RT \ln (C_2/C_1)/\omega^2 (1-vp) (d_2^2 - d_1^2)$$

with C_1 and C_2 = concentrations of particles at d_1 and d_2 distances from the axis of rotation, ω = angular velocity, v = partial specific volume, and p = density of solution. Centrifugation is continued until the concentration of particles is in a steady state.

Based on the work of W. J. Archibald in 1947, a variation on the sedimentation equilibrium method was developed. This is called *approach to equilibrium* and takes advantage of the fact that the solute at the meniscus and bottom of a cell are in equilibrium. As the equation describing this situation is the same as that for complete equilibrium, it is possible to determine the molecular weight. The net result is a molecular weight determined after a short centrifuge run at low speed.

ROTORS

The heart of the centrifuge technique, the rotor, is generally designed for either preparative or analytical purposes. The preparative rotors are either of the angle, swinging-bucket, or zonal type. The angle rotors consist of cavities in a solid support at an angle to the axis of rotation into which containers made of various materials are placed. The swinging-bucket apparatus consists of a bucket freely held by pins into which a container is placed. At rest, the bucket is parallel to the axis of rotation, but during movement, centrifugal force pulls it into a perpendicular position. Finally, zonal rotors usually have hollow, sector-shaped compartments perpendicular to the axis of rotation. The gradient may be introduced while the rotor spins along with the sample. The high speed possible allows better separation of particles in distinct zones according to density or size.

Centrifuges used for analytical purposes are usually made so that light may pass through the cells of the material being examined and thereby determine the solute boundary position. This is achieved through an optical system which measures the absorption or refraction.

DENSITY GRADIENT CENTRIFUGATION

Density gradient centrifugation uses a solution that increases in density down through the container. There are basically two types: zonal and *isopycnic.* Zonal density gradient centrifugation, or velocity centrifugation as it is sometimes called, involves a preformed gradient, usually of sucrose, produced by mixing a sucrose and water solution in layers for a continuous gradient, or in pipetted layers of decreasing density on top of each other for a discontinuous gradient. The sample mixture is placed on top of the gradient in the tube and allowed to sediment at different rates according to the particular macromolecule. This technique takes a short period of time, the mixture separating according to size, shape, and density until equilibrium is reached the sedimentation coefficient can then be determined according to where the bands are located.

In isopycnic or equilibrium density gradient centrifugation, the separation of particles is based on density differences alone. The sample is mixed in a solution – usually cesium chloride ($CsCl$), because of its high solubility and low viscosity – and is spun for a long period of time (sometimes days). The $CsCl$ sediments to form a gradient and the macromolecules band at those points where their density equals that of the $CsCl$ with high resolution.

With either type of density gradient centrifugation, the sedimentation coefficient may be determined by comparing the known sedimentation coefficient of one macromolecule to an unknown. The two macromolecules are sedimented together and the relationship

$$s_{20,w} \text{ (unknown)} = s_{20,w} \text{ (standard) } \frac{d \text{ (unknown)}}{d \text{ (standard)}}$$

is used, with d (unknown) and d (standard) equaling distance traveled by each macromolecule band from the meniscus.

BIBLIOGRAPHY

Collowick, S. P., and Kaplan, N. O. (Eds.) *Methods in Enzymology.* New York: Academic, 1957. Vol. 4.
Chervenka, C. H. *A Manual of Methods for the Analytical Ultracentrifuge.* Palo Alto, California: Beckman Instruments, 1969.
Debuve, C., Barlthet, J., and Beaufay, H. Gradient centrifugation of cell particles. Theory and applications. *Prog. Biophys. Chem.* 9:325, 1959.

IV   Chromatography

One of the most common laboratory problems is the separation, or at least detection of the presence of, different chemicals in a mixture. One of the very important methods of doing this is partition chromatography. It is a two-phase system, essentially based on the distribution of different chemicals between two solvents that do not mix. A long glass column is fitted in the bottom with a glass filter, or a little glass wool, and is filled with an inert powder suspended in a solvent. Most of the solvent will go through, leaving behind the column of powder retaining some solvent in its pores.

The sample is then poured in through the top, followed by the second solvent. As this second solvent goes through the column, it carries down the chemicals from the sample. Small fractions of the liquid that come down are collected in a test tube. A fraction collector can be used which automatically changes tubes, either collecting fixed volumes of liquid or changing tubes at fixed intervals of time.

The process can be imagined as being divided into a number of discrete steps. In each step the chemicals will distribute themselves between mobile and stationary phases according to their relative solubility in each solvent. Consider a substance that dissolves equally well in each solvent (it is considered as having a partition coefficient of 1). In the first step the substance will be in the first layer. Then half will move down, with the solvent, to a second layer. As more solvent comes in, half the substance from the second layer will move to the third layer, and half from the first layer to the second layer. This process will go on, and after a number of times the chemical will be concentrated in a narrow band somewhere in the column (Fig. IV-1).

If a second chemical with a partition coefficient of 0.5 is mixed in the sample, it will layer above the first one and be completely separate from it. Both chemicals will move down and can be collected separately.

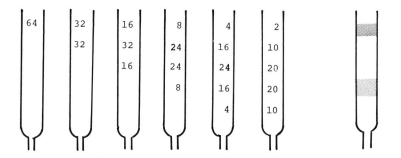

Fig. IV-1. Partition chromatography.

A filter paper can be used instead of the column. The samples are applied to the paper as very small spots. The paper is then put into a glass jar, with the solvent but not touching it, and allowed to equilibrate with the solvent vapors. Generally a water-immiscible solvent saturated with water is used. A cellulose filter paper will take up moisture, and will constitute a water-stationary phase. The paper is then put in contact with the solvent. If the solvent is in the bottom of the jar, it rises through the paper and the process is called *ascending chromatography*. If the solvent is in a container on the top, it descends, and the process is called *descending chromatography* (Fig. IV-2). As the solvent travels up or down through the paper, the chemicals separate in spots.

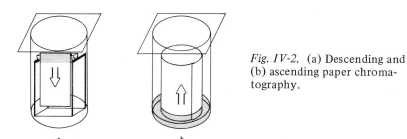

Fig. IV-2. (a) Descending and (b) ascending paper chromatography.

If the chemicals are colorless, the paper can be sprayed with the proper reagents to produce colored spots. In some cases ultraviolet lamps may be used to examine the paper, as certain chemicals absorb ultraviolet and will appear as black spots against a violet background. Other chemicals are strongly fluorescent under ultraviolet light.

Chromatographs should be run at a constant temperature, as temperature changes may even change the distribution coefficient. They are therefore carried out in places removed from sources of heat or cold, and drafts, if possible, in a controlled temperature environment.

The migration of samples is expressed as the ratio of the distance traveled by each spot to the distance the solvent migrates to. This is called R_f.

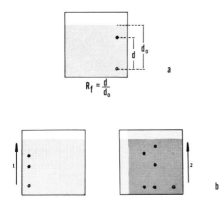

$$R_f = \frac{d}{d_0}$$

Fig. IV-3. (a) One-dimensional and (b) two-dimensional chromatography. Blank circle is starting point of sample's migration.

When there is a mixture of many components of similar structure, generally one solvent will not separate all the components. Two solvents can then be run in sequence. After the first run is done, the paper is turned at right angles and the second solvent is run. This is called *bidimensional chromatography.* Still another chromatographic method involves putting the suspension of the supporting material in a glass plate. Generally the supporting material is mixed with gypsum, and when a slurry of the mixture is applied to glass it will form a firm coating. Already-coated pieces of plastic or glass now exist. The plate is then put into a jar, touching the solvent, as with paper chromatography. This is called *thin-layer chromatography.*

In the case of substances poorly soluble in water, a filter paper made of glass fiber is used, so that the stationary phase is a nonaqueous solvent. Water can then be the mobile phase. This is called *reverse chromatography.*

With all three techniques — column, thin-layer, and paper chromatography — the principle is *partition* between two immiscible solvents. But this is not the only mechanism for separation. Even with two immiscible liquids and an inert support, other factors may be active. One is the *adsorption* of the chemicals in the support. By weak chemical forces, the chemicals may attach themselves to the surface of the support and then be removed (eluted) by the mobile phase. When this mechanism occurs, frequently the chemical cannot be extracted from the column unless a different solvent from the one in which it was introduced washes the column. If the chemical was introduced as a water solution, it may be eluted only in a solution of different salt concentration or different pH. Several materials which absorb chemicals well are used to make the column (e.g., silicic acid, alumina, infusoria earth).

A third basic mechanism of separation is *ion exchange*. The column in this case contains a large polymer, with weak acidic or basic groups. The substances to be separated may react with these groups and be retained as salts. When the column is washed with an acid or basic solvent, the chemicals are displaced, emerging with the solvent. Different chemicals will emerge at different fractions, as their equilibrium constant is different, and will be displaced either at different times or only with stronger concentrations of solvent. These materials are called *ion-exchange resins*.

Still another separation mechanism is supplied by polymers in small beads, with varying sizes of pores. Small molecules can cross the pores inside the small beads. Large molecules are excluded and will come through the column with the initial solvent, according to their size, the largest molecules being eluted first. When more solvent is added, the small molecules are washed out. Materials are now available with ranges of pores for separating materials of different molecular sizes. They can even be used to estimate the size of the molecules (molecular weight and shape enter into the determination of the size of molecules). This is called *gel filtration*.

BIBLIOGRAPHY

Determann, H. *Gel Chromatography.* New York: Springer, 1969.
Stahl, E. *Thin Layer Chromatography* (2nd ed.). New York: Springer, 1969.

V   pH, Titration, and Buffers

IONIZATION OF WATER

Water dissociates according to the equation

$$H_2O \rightleftharpoons H^+ + OH^-$$

The hydrogen ion, however, is not stable as a proton, and it therefore associates with another water molecule to form a hydroxonium ion. Thus the dissociation of water is

$$2H_2O \rightleftharpoons OH_3^+ + OH^-$$

although usually we continue to speak of hydrogen ions. The equilibrium equation for the dissociation can be written in the form:

$$K = \frac{(H^+)(OH^-)}{(H_2O)} \text{ or } K_w = K(H_2O) = (H^+)(OH^-)$$

In dilute solutions the concentration of water is practically constant ($1000/18 = 55.5M$). At $25°$ C (room temperature) $K_w = 10^{14}$.

In pure water the concentrations of H^+ and OH^- are equal. So $(H^+) = (OH^-) = 10^{-7}M$. If we add hydrogen ions (by adding an acid) the excess H^+ will combine with OH^- until the product of the concentration goes back to 10^{-14}. Therefore each time (H^+) goes up, (OH^-) goes down.

(H^+)	(OH^-)	pH
$1M = 10^0 M$	$10^{-14}M$	0
$0.1M = 10^{-1}M$	$10^{-13}M$	1
$10^{-2}M$	$10^{-12}M$	2
$10^{-3}M$	$10^{-11}M$	3
$10^{-4}M$	$10^{-10}M$	4
$10^{-5}M$	$10^{-9}M$	5
$10^{-6}M$	$10^{-8}M$	6
$10^{-7}M$	$10^{-7}M$	7
$10^{-8}M$	$10^{-6}M$	8
$10^{-9}M$	$10^{-5}M$	9
$10^{-10}M$	$10^{-4}M$	10
$10^{-11}M$	$10^{-3}M$	11
$10^{-12}M$	$10^{-2}M$	12
$10^{-13}M$	$10^{-1}M$	13
$10^{-14}M$	$10^{-0}M$	14

To avoid having to handle small concentrations, the log $1/(H^+)$ is used. This is called the *pH*.

$$(H^+)(OH^-) = 10^{-14}$$

$$\log 1/(H^+) + \log 1/(OH^-) = \log 10^{14}$$

$$pH + pOH = 14$$

pH is an expression for the hydrogen ion concentration, corrected for interaction between ions. (We are not always dealing with very dilute solutions.)

At $25°C$, pH = pOH = 7. This point is called the *neutral point*. When the pH is lower, the solution is acidic; when higher, alkaline. pH 7 is frequently considered to be the neutral point, even at other temperatures. At $37°C$ (the human body's normal temperature), pH 6.8 is the neutral point.

DETERMINATION OF pH

It has been found that a certain kind of glass is pH-sensitive. A very thin tube is made of this glass and is filled with $0.1M$ hydrochloric acid. A silver wire is then introduced into the tube. This arrangement is called a glass electro

When the electrode is introduced into a solution, it acquires a potential proportional to the external pH. An absolute potential cannot be measured. The glass electrode is connected to a standard electrode, forming a cell. The potential difference of this cell depends on the pH into which the glass electrode is dipped.

A commonly used standard electrode is made by introducing a platinum wire into a mixture of mercury (mercurous chloride, or calomel) and saturated potassium chloride solution. A small hole establishes communication between the external solution and the saturated potassium chloride.

The two electrodes form a battery which has an emf (voltage) proportional to the pH of the solution into which it is dipped. The emf is measured with a voltmeter especially designed for potentials across high resistances (the glass wall of the glass electrode has a high resistance) and is graduated directly in pH units. This instrument is called a pH meter.

To calibrate a pH meter, a solution of known pH is used as a standard (a good one is $20M$ potassium acid phthalate, which has a pH of 4). The electrodes are immersed in this solution, and the instrument is set by turning of the calibration dial to the known pH. The solution is then removed, and the electrodes are washed with distilled water and inserted in the unknown solution. The pH is then read directly.

The glass and calomel electrodes vary with the potential as the temperature changes. To avoid lengthy calculation, pH meters have a dial graduated for temperature range. The temperature of the solution should be set on the meter before calibration. It is important also that both the standard and the solution be at the same temperature.

The electrodes need proper care if exact readings are to be obtained. Electrodes should never be allowed to dry but should be kept in water at all times. The potential of the reference electrode depends on the concentration of potassium chloride. The solution should be kept saturated by adding more potassium chloride crystals when needed. The glass electrode is very thin and breaks easily. (If this happens, the pH will always close to 3.) The glass may also combine with proteins, heavy metals, and other impurities from solutions used. This makes it lose its sensitivity, preventing it from reacting to pH changes. In some cases, washing the glass overnight in $1M$ hydrochloric acid may reactivate the electrode.

TITRATION OF A STRONG ACID

Hydrochloric acid is a strong acid. All its molecules are dissociated into the chloride and hydrogen ions, and its pH is approximately 1. If 10 ml of $1.0M$

hydrochloric acid is put into a beaker, and concentrated sodium hydroxide added to it, the substances will combine, removing the hydrogen ions.

$$H^+ + Cl^- + Na^+ + OH^- \rightleftharpoons H_2O + Na^+ + Cl^-$$

When enough sodium hydroxide is added to neutralize 90 percent of the acid, the concentration will be close to $0.1M$ and the pH equal to 2. When 99 percent of the acid is neutralized, the pH will go up to 3, and if it were possible to stop at 99.9 percent, the pH would be 3. In reality it is difficult to stop at this point, as a drop of sodium hydroxide will neutralize all the acid, and the excess sodium hydroxide will raise the pH above 8.

TITRATION OF A WEAK ACID

If the titration is started with a weak acid such as acetic acid, only a small proportion of the molecules are ionized.

$$\frac{(H^+) (CH_3COO^-)}{(CH_3COOH)} = 1.74 \times 0.10^{-5}M$$

The initial pH is about 3, and the change of pH with the concentration is regulated as shown by Figure V-1.

Upon addition of the first drops of sodium hydroxide there is a large change in pH. Then it changes very slowly until most of the acid reacts with the hydroxide. In the middle of the reaction there is a mixture of acetic acid, mostly not dissociated, and sodium acetate, mostly dissociated:

$$CH_3COOH \rightleftharpoons H^+ + CH_3COO^-$$

$$Na^+ + CH_3COO^-$$

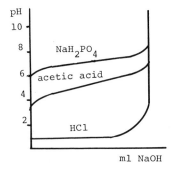

Fig. V-1. pH change during titration.

This solution (containing a weak acid and its salt) is called a *buffer,* and it is a solution that resists pH changes. If sodium hydroxide is added to a mixture of acetic acid and acetate, OH^+ combines with H^+, forming water. As this occurs, more acetic acid molecules dissociate, restoring the H^+ concentration. If an acid is added instead of a base, the excess H^+ combines with CH_3COO^- to form acetic acid, restoring the pH.

We can write

$$K = \frac{(H^+)\,(CH_3COO^-)}{(CH_3COOH)} \quad \text{or}$$

$$(H^+) = K\,\frac{(CH_3COOH)}{(CH_3COO^-)} \quad \text{or}$$

$$-\log(H^+) = -\log K - \log\frac{(CH_3COOH)}{(CH_3COO^-)}$$

replacing $-\log(H^+)$ by pH, and $-\log K$ by pK

$$pH = pK + \log\frac{(CH_3COO^-)}{(CH_3COOH)}$$

where the acetate ion concentration is practically the same as the concentration of acetate salt present. As most of the acid is not dissociated, and acetic acid, we can say that

$$pH = pK + \log\frac{salt}{acid}$$

When the concentrations of salt and acid are equal, the ratio of the two is 1, and $\log 1 = 0$, so we have pH = pK. Therefore pK can be measured from pH when half the acid is neutralized. It is clear now that, as more sodium hydroxide is added, the concentration of salt goes up whereas acid concentration goes down, and pH changes more and more rapidly. The reverse occurs when acid is added, with the salt concentration going down and the acid concentration up.

In order to keep a solution at a certain pH, buffers are added. The buffer selected must have a pK close to the pH to be maintained. Observe on the graph (Fig. V–1) the buffer effect of NaH_2PO_4.

A MORE GENERAL CONCEPT OF ACIDS

Lowry and Bornsted called an acid any molecule that could donate proteins On losing protons, it is transformed into a *conjugated base* which may take protons back.

Water can be either an acid or a base, as on dissociation one molecule is the acid and the other the base.

$$H_2O + H_2O \rightleftharpoons OH_3^+ + OH^-$$

$$acid_1 + base_2 \rightleftharpoons acid_2 + base_1$$

The reaction always involves a transfer of protons to a second base that become an acid.

$$HCl + H_2O \rightleftharpoons OH_3^+ + Cl^-$$

$$acid_1 + base_2 \rightleftharpoons acid_2 + base_1$$

Similarly we can call

$$CH_3COOH + NaOH \rightleftharpoons CH_3COO^- + H_2O + Na^+$$

$$\quad acid_1 \qquad base_2 \qquad\qquad base_1 \qquad acid_2$$

and

$$NaH_2PO_4 + NaOH \rightleftharpoons Na_2HCO_4 + H_2O$$

$$\quad acid_1 \qquad base_2 \qquad\qquad base_1 \qquad acid_2$$

giving the general equation

$$pH = pK + \log \frac{(base)}{(acid)}$$

This is called the Henderson-Hasselbalch equation.

VI   Probability and Statistics

When you toss a coin, it can fall either heads up or tails up. Neither one of the two possibilities is more likely than the other, and therefore the probability that heads will fall up should be half the time you toss the coin. The probability of each result per toss is 1/2.

If you toss the same coin twice, there are four possibilities: heads-heads, heads-tails, tails-heads, or tails-tails. The probability of getting heads the first time is 1/2; the probability is also 1/2 the second time, since the second throw is independent of the first. The probability of obtaining heads twice is 1/2 × 1/2, or 1/4, that is, 1 chance in 4. The probability is the same for getting tails-tails, heads-tails, or tails-heads. If two identical coins are tossed at the same time, there is no particular order to the results obtained, since two heads-and-tails combinations occur at the same time. In this case, the probability of having one heads and one tails is the sum of the probabilities for the ordered combinations, 1/4 + 1/4 = 1/2.

To find probabilities for more than two coins, we use the Pascal triangle, named for the famous seventeenth-century mathematician who began the study of probability:

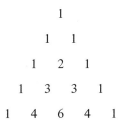

where each number is the sum of the two numbers to the left and right above it. We can use this triangle to find the probabilities of various combinations of heads and tails. For instance, in three tosses, there are eight possibilities (HHH, HHT, HTH, THH, TTH, THT, HTT, and TTT). There is 1 chance in 8 for all tails, and the same for all heads, 3/8 for two tails and one head (in any order and 3/8 for two heads and one tail. The sum of numbers in the fourth row of Pascal's triangle $(1 + 3 + 3 + 1)$ is 8. If we let the numbers represent ratios $(1:3:3:1)$, we see that they correspond to the ratios just given: 1 (all heads): 3 (one head + two tails): 3 (two heads + one tail): 1 (all tails). This demonstrates the usefulness of Pascal's triangle. In this discussion, two things are implicitly assumed: (1) for any toss, the chance of getting a head is equal to that of getting a tail, and (2) each individual toss is independent of every other toss.

Another method of deriving the numbers in Pascal's triangle is to calculate the numerical coefficients of the polynomial $(p + q)^n$, which will give us the numbers for the nth horizontal line of Pascal's triangle. For example, if $n = 3$, we have

$$(p + q)^n = (p + q)^3$$

$$= p^3 + 3p^2q + 3pq^2 + q^3$$

Taking the coefficients in order gives line three of Pascal's triangle as 1, 3, 3, 1. Note further that if we let p = probability of tossing a head = 1/2 and q = probability of tossing a tail = 1/2, then we can calculate the probabilities of the vario combinations of heads and tails we could get from three tosses of a coin (or, similarly, the simultaneous tossing of three coins):

1. $p^3 = (1/2)^3 = 1/8$, the probability for three consecutive heads

2. $3p^2 q = 3 (1/2)^2 (1/2) = 3 (1/2)^3 = 3/8$, the probability for two heads and one tail

Calculation of the probability of three tails, or of two tails and one head is done similarly.

Suppose now we have a box which contains two white balls and one black ball. If a ball is drawn from the box at random, the probability of drawing a white ball, p, is 2/3; the probability of drawing a black ball, q, is 1/3. Suppose four drawings are made, the result recorded each time, and the ball that was drawn then placed back in the box. We can use the polynomial $(p + q)^4$ to calculate the probabilities of drawing various combinations of black and white balls, in a manner similar to the previous case with the coins:

$$(p + q)^4 = (p^2 + 2pq + q^2)^2$$

$$= p^4 + 4p^3q + 6p^2q^2 + 4pq^3 + q^4$$

Thus,

p^4 = probability of drawing only white balls

= 16/81

$4p^3q$ = probability of drawing three whites and one black

= 32/81

$6p^2q^2$ = probability of drawing two whites and one black

= 24/81

$4pq^3$ = probability of drawing one white and three blacks

= 8/81

q^4 = probability of drawing only black balls

= 1/81

Note that the sum of all these probabilities equals 1, as expected.

Going back to coin tosses and Pascal's triangle, notice that, for the case of n = 3, it is three times more likely to get a combination of heads and tails than to get only heads or only tails. For, say, n = 4, it is 4 times more probable to get 3 heads and one tail than 4 tails, and one and one-half times more probable to get three heads and two tails than four heads and one tail. This distribution is demonstrated in the histogram of Figure VI-1.

Extrapolating this argument to increasingly larger numbers of tosses, it is clear that the likelihood of having approximately the same number of heads and tails is greater than the likelihood of having an excess of one over the other. This is essentially a restatement of the fact that, on each throw, either heads or tails may appear with equal likelihood. Thus, in throwing a coin many times, one would expect equal numbers of heads and tails. If a histogram

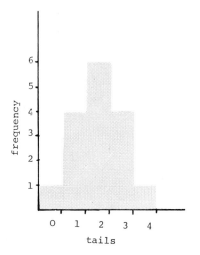

Fig. VI-1. Heads and tails distribution for four coins.

similar to that of Figure VI-1 is drawn for large n, it begins to approximate the bell-shaped curve shown in Figure VI-2.

This figure represents what is referred to as a *normal distribution.* The peak of the curve occurs at the expected value of the measured characteristic. For instance, if the ratio of heads to tails is measured in a large number of tosses, the peak of the curve lies above the value 1. Note that this represents a continuous distribution of values around x̄ and thus can only approximate the discontinuous values seen in Figure VI-1. Whereas from the histogram we can

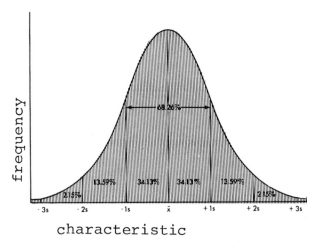

Fig. VI-2. Normal distribution.

determine the probability of a particular, unique event (such as five heads, or three heads and two tails), when the normal distribution is used, we ask the question, "What is the probability that a particular measurement lies within two specified values?" The question is answered by calculating the area under the curve within the values specified. (The total area under the curve, which represents all possible outcomes of the specified experiment, must equal 1.) Thus, in Figure VI-2, $\bar{x}$ represents the expected value, or mean, of a measured characteristic. For example, the outcome of an experiment which has an expected value of $\bar{x}$ will lie within 1s (one standard deviation) of $\bar{x}$ 68.26 percent of the time. The value of $\bar{x}$ depends, of course, on what is being measured, and the meaning and calculation of s is explained below.

MEANS AND STANDARD DEVIATION

Since some results deviate to the right and others to the left (these results are numerical values), a mean will cancel the deviations:

$$\bar{x} = \frac{\Sigma \, (\text{value})}{n}$$

where $\bar{x}$ is the mean, Σ indicates a sum, and n represents the number of values.

The mean, frequently used to express the best value, does not give an additional important piece of information: the spread of the results (the *distribution*). This spread tells how the individual results vary, what the chance is that these results are close to the theoretical value, and where the mean will most likely be found if the experiment is repeated.

To provide this information, without presenting each individual result (in some experiments there might be hundreds or thousands of observations), it is customary to calculate the *standard deviation* (s). This value is found by the formula

$$s^2 = \frac{\Sigma \, (\text{measures})^2 - 1/n \, (\Sigma \, \text{measures})^2}{n - 1}$$

where n = number of results.

If a very large number of measurements are made, 68.3 percent of the results come out within the range of the mean $\pm$s and 99.7 percent within the range of the mean $\pm$3s. A value outside the range of the mean $\pm$3s has only 3 chances in 1,000 of being close to the theoretical value.

Results are frequently expressed as either the mean ± s or the mean ± $s/\sqrt{n}$ (the standard error). Of course, the standard error decreases as the number of observations increases.

t TEST

Imagine that you have two sets of data (e.g., measurements of some experiment), each set with a normal distribution, and you want to find out if the two sets belong to the same population of data. The assumption that they do indeed belong together is called the *null hypothesis,* and it is frequently used in analysis of experiments. For example, if two groups of animals are being used to test for the effects of a vitamin, the data from the test group and from the control group must be analyzed to see if there is a significant difference between them. The *t* test will show what the probability is that the two sets are not different.

The means and the standard deviations for the sets a and b are calculated, and from these and the number of data in each set (n), the value for *t* is found by using the formula

$$t = \frac{\bar{x}_a - \bar{x}_b}{\sqrt{\dfrac{s_a{}^2}{n_a} + \dfrac{s_b{}^2}{n_b}}}$$

where $\bar{x}_a$ is always the larger of the two means.

By using the *t* table (Table VI-1), one can find the probability that the data sets are similar. The degree of freedom (df) = $n_a + n_b - 2$. Locate, on the *t* table, the df appropriate for the data sets, and look at the numbers in the columns to the right of it. For example, assume df = 10. If the value for t is greater than or equal to 1.81, there is a 0.1 probability (1 chance in 10) that the data sets are not significantly different (or 9 chances in 10 that the data sets *are* significantly different). If the value for $t \geqslant 2.23$, there is a 0.05 probability (5 chances in 100) that the data sets are *not* significantly different (or 95 chances in 100 that the data sets *are* significantly different). The procedure is similar for 0.01 and 0.001 probabilities. A probability of 0.05 or smaller indicates that it is highly probable that the two sets of data are similar.

CHI-SQUARE TEST

If you toss a coin a hundred times, you would expect fifty heads and fifty tails. If you get 36/64, can you assume that either the coin is asymmetrical or

Table VI-1. Values of *t*

df	Probability			
	0.1	0.05	0.01	0.001
1	6.31	12.71	63.66	636.62
2	2.92	4.30	9.93	31.60
3	2.35	3.18	5.84	12.94
4	2.13	2.77	4.60	8.61
5	2.01	2.57	4.03	6.86
6	1.94	2.45	3.71	5.96
7	1.89	2.36	3.50	5.40
8	1.86	2.31	3.36	5.04
9	1.83	2.26	3.25	4.78
10	1.81	2.23	3.17	4.59
12	1.78	2.18	3.06	4.32
14	1.76	2.14	2.98	4.14
17	1.74	2.11	2.90	3.97
20	1.73	2.09	2.85	3.85
25	1.71	2.06	2.79	3.73
30	1.70	2.04	2.75	3.65
60	1.67	2.00	2.70	3.55
120	1.66	1.98	2.62	3.37
∞	1.65	1.96	2.56	3.29

that you are tossing with a bias? This is typical of cases in which statistical methods are employed to compare experimental data with expected data.

In the statistical test a value called *chi-square* is calculated:

$$\chi^2 = \Sigma \ \frac{(\text{observed} - \text{expected})^2}{\text{expected}}$$

For the coin example, χ^2 is 7.84. This χ^2 relates the probability of finding the experimental data to the proposed theoretical expectation (50/50). In the chi-square test, df = number of classes of data-independent variables. In the coin example, the number of classes = 2 (heads, tails), and the number of dependent variables = 1 (arbitrarily either heads or tails; e.g., the appearance of tails depends on whether heads lands up). For most data, the dependent variables = 1, but in some complex cases, the number may be greater than 1.

For a χ^2 of 7.84, find the appropriate df (1) in Table VI-2 and read to the right. This gives χ^2 corresponding to a probability of between 0.01 and 0.001. This means that the experimental result will occur between 0.1 and 1 times in 100, or that the data obtained can be expected to occur by chance alone

Table VI-2. Chi-Square

			Probability			
df	0.9	0.5	0.2	0.05	0.01	0.001
1	.02	.46	1.64	3.84	6.63	10.83
2	.21	1.39	3.22	5.99	9.21	13.82
3	.58	2.37	4.64	7.82	11.35	16.27
4	1.06	3.37	5.99	9.49	13.27	18.47
5	1.61	4.35	7.29	11.07	15.09	20.52
6	2.20	5.35	8.56	12.59	16.82	22.46
7	2.83	6.35	9.80	14.07	18.47	24.32
8	3.49	7.35	11.30	15.51	20.10	26.12
9	4.17	8.34	12.24	16.92	21.67	26.88
10	4.86	9.34	13.44	18.31	23.21	29.56

between 1 percent and 0.1 percent of the time. For a small number of results and 1 degree of freedom, the calculation of chi-square is corrected to

$$\chi^2 = \Sigma \ \frac{(\text{observed} - \text{expected}) - 0.5)^2}{\text{expected}}$$

HOMOGENEITY TEST

In a group of children, imagine that there appears to be a 1:1 ratio of normal to abnormal children. To test whether the proportion of normal to abnormal changes with sex, a table can be drawn up on the assumption that both groups belong to the same homogeneous sample, with an expected ratio of 1:1.

Sex	Observed or Expected	Normal	Abnormal	Total	χ^2	df	P
Male	Obs.	30	36	66	0.54	1	0.2−0.5
	Exp.	33	33				
Female	Obs.	42	30	72	2.00	1	0.05−0.2
	Exp.	36	36				
Total group	Obs.	72	66	138	0.26	1	0.5−0.9
	Exp.	69	69				
adding χ^2 of separate groups					2.54	2	0.2−0.5
difference between χ^2 of separate groups and χ^2 of total group					2.28	1	0.05−0.2

It can therefore be concluded, from the χ^2 of the difference (calculated above), that the probability that the two groups (males, females) will be different is between 0.05 and 0.2 or, by interpolation, close to 0.1.

CONTINGENCY TABLES

In the homogeneity test, we took an assumption (that the normal/abnormal character was independent of sex) and calculated the expected ratio of normal to abnormal characteristics. When it is a question of two alternative characteristics that need to be related to two conditions (like the relationship of sex, to mild and strong forms of a disease or to infection or lack of infection), it is difficult to predict an expected result. In this case a 2 x 2 table (contingency table) can be used:

Characteristic

Condition	With	Without	Total
A	a	b	n_1
B	c	d	n_2
A + B	n_3	n_4	N

The tabulated data can be analyzed by the formula

$$\chi^2 = \frac{[(a \cdot d) - (b \cdot c)]^2 \, N}{n_1 \cdot n_2 \cdot n_3 \cdot n_4}$$

This χ^2 is treated just like the previous χ^2 (see chi-square test), and has similar implications.

STRAIGHT LINE

When data is plotted, the points often have a linear relationship, that is, they all lie more or less on a straight line. This relationship can be very useful in predicting values between or beyond the points determined experimentally.

The general equation for a line is $y = a + bx$, where a is the y-intercept (when $x = 0$), and b is the slope of the line, generally determined by $b = (x_2 - x_1)/(y_2 - y_1)$.

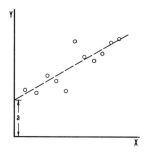

Fig. VI-3. Regression.

In order to give the best possible equation and draw the best possible line, each experimental data point should deviate as little as possible from the line. To accomplish this, the method of least squares can be used to find a and b:

$$b = \frac{\Sigma \, (\overline{x} - x) \, (\overline{y} - y)}{\Sigma \, (\overline{x} - x)^2}$$

and $a = y - bx$

The summation is done for all x and y in the experimental data. A graph can then be drawn from these calculated slope and intercept values which will be better than one drawn from the experimental x and y values.

VII   Answers to the Self-Evaluation Tests

Chapter 1

1: b
2: d
3: a
4: b
5: c
6: a

Chapter 2

1: Ala–Phe–Arg–His–Leu–Phe–Leu
2: c
3: a
4: b
5: b
6: d
7: d
8: a

Chapter 3

1.a: t 1.b: q 1.c: s 1.d: p
2.a: p 2.b: s 2.c: q
3.a: p 3.b: r 3.c: p, v 3.d: q, t
4.a: q, v, x 4.b: p, s, y 4.c: r, u, v or w
5: d
6.a: q, r 6.b: s 6.c: p

Chapter 4

1.a: r   1.b: u   1.c: r
2: a
3.a: q   3.b: p   3.c: r
4: b
5: 200/16

Chapter 5

1. S: GAG by GUA
   C: GAG by AAG
   E: GAG by AAG
   Memphis: GAG by CAG

2. G:C pairs share three hydrogen bonds, whereas A:T pairs share two. Thus, DNA with a higher G:C content has, in effect, more hydrogen bonds holding it together, thus requiring more heat to cause the strands to separate.

3. Arg, Ser, Gly, Phe, Leu, Tyr, and termination.

4. Crossing-over leads to segregation of genes that are linked on the same chromosomes; sister exchange has no genetic consequences.

5. The primer provides the beginning for chain growth, and the template provides the information for the sequence being synthesized.

6. To repair DNA split by enzymes such as endonucleases; to eliminate portions of the chain that must be repaired after damage caused by ultraviolet radiation or ionizing radiations; to seal the small segments produced in the process of DNA replication.

7. There would be two mRNAs for a single gene, resulting in two different proteins, according to the sequence of the nucleotides.

8. ATP is used in the synthesis of aminoacyl-tRNA, and GTP for the elongation of the chain.

9. The codon for methionine for initiation, and the three nonsense codons for termination.

10. Actinomycin D binds to DNA, preventing transcription. Cycloheximide and chloramphenicol block protein synthesis, the first in eukaryotes, and the second in prokaryotes and mitochondria of eukaryotes.

11. DNA replication occurs in the nucleus, in the mitochondria, and possibly in other parts of the cell as well. Ribosomal synthesis occurs in the nucleoli.

12. The entire message is misread. Sometimes activity can be partially restored by a nearby insertion of a nucleotide, thus throwing the message off only in the region between the deletion and the insertion.

13. One conclusive experiment would be competitive hybridization. Hybridize 28S RNA to ribosomal DNA, to saturation. Now add labeled 18S RNA, and determine the amount of label which hybridizes to the DNA. Repeat without the 28S RNA present. If the levels of label hybridized to the rDNA genes are the same, this shows that 28S and 18S RNA do not compete for the same sites on the DNA, and therefore do not have similar nucleotide sequences.

Chapter 6

1. The law applies to a population in which mating (in relation to the genes under consideration) occurs at random. It predicts that, if two alleles are in equilibrium, the frequency of the alleles will not change.

2. The frequency of the allele in the rest of the population is $1:3$, so that in the next generation 0.33×0.33, or $.1089$, of the population will be homozygous for this gene.

3. a. The population is not mating at random (due to social, racial, or religious groups that do not intermarry).
   b. The character under consideration is discriminated against in mating.
   c. The pressure of selection is either against the homozygote or for the heterozygote.

4. b, c.

Index

Abnormal children, percentage
of, 195
Acetabularia
experiment of Hammerling, 120,
122, 123
study of Brachet and Chantrene,
153
Acetic acid, 38
titration of, 234–235
Acid-acetone treatment, in preparation of globin, 18
Acids
general concept of, 236
titration of, 233–235
Acridine, in testing genetic code,
177
Acriflavine, structure of, 178
Acrylamide gel, in disc electrophoresis, 221
Actinomycin, blocking effects of
erythropoietin, 182
Actinomycin D, in study of RNA,
160, 161
Adenine, structure of, 120, 127
Absorption, as mechanism in chromatography, 229–230
African Negro tribes, and sickle-cell
trait, 199
Alanine, chemical formula of, 34
Albinism, 152
Alkaptonuria, 152
Alleles, 77
and variations in hereditary traits,
96
Alpha chains, of hemoglobin
molecule, 23, 27

blocked production in thalassemia,
54
Alpha helix, of polypeptide chain,
32, 33
Altitudes, high
and blood hemoglobin content, 41
and red blood cell production, 49
Amino acids
incorporation into proteins, 163
mass of, 27
and proteins, 17, 18, 24, 25
replacement in abnormal hemoglobin chain, 86
separation from protein hydrolyzate,
quantitative method of Moore
and Stein, 24
sequence of, 114
structure of, 23–31, 34
substitutions of, 37
in thin-layer chromatography, 19, 20
Amish, Older Order of, genetic
anomaly among, 189
Amniotic cavity, puncturing of, and
detection of hereditary
disease, 196
Amoebas, and microsurgery, Goldstein
and Plaut studies, 153
Analgesics, and aplastic anemia, 50
Anemia(s), 48–52
aplastic, agents producing, 50
causes of, 47, 49
defined, 48
diagnosis of, laboratory investigation, 52–53
experimental, laboratory investigation, 48

Anemia(s) – *Continued*
 hemolytic, susceptibility as
  hereditary trait, 97
 iron deficiency, 50–51
 pernicious, 52
 primaquine, 100
 sickle-cell, 54
  coinciding with sickle-cell trait,
   199
  criteria for, 79
  and genetic counseling, 85
  surveying for presence of, 82, 83
Anopheles gambiae mosquitoes, in
  sickle-cell experiments, 202
Antibiotics
 and aplastic anemia, 50
 as inhibitors of protein synthesis,
  172
Anticodon, 179, 180
Anticonvulsants, and aplastic
  anemia, 50
Antimalarial drugs
 and metabolic defects in anemia,
  55
 and susceptibility to hemolytic
  anemia, 97
Apoferritin, 51
Ascaris cells, and meiosis, 115–116
Ascorbic acid, combining with iron,
  50

Banding, of macromolecules in
  ultracentrifuge, 141, 142
Barth's hemoglobin, 54
Beadle and Tatum, "one gene-one
  enzyme" theory of, 153
Beans, broad. *See Vicia faba*
Benzene, and aplastic anemia, 50
Beta chains, of hemoglobin
  molecule, 23, 27
 blocked production in thalassemia, 54
Bilroth cords, 49
Birth defects, lowering rate of, 197
Bleeders. *See* Hemophilia
Blood
 loss of, as cause of anemia, 49, 51
 sample, procedures for obtaining,
  2, 4
 venous, migration of ions, 11
Blood plasma, measurement of molecule and ion concentration, 6

Blood smear, preparation of, 4
Bohr effect, 40
 and anemia, 54
Boiling point, of solutions, 6
Bone marrow
 abnormal, diagnosis of, 50
 in production of red blood cells, 48
Bragg, and effects of X-rays on
  crystal, 31
Brazil, percent of first-cousin
  marriages, 191
Buffer solution, 235
 and electrophoretic mobility,
  219–220

Carbamino groups, in carbon dioxide
  transport, 43
Carbon dioxide transport, role of
  hemoglobin in, 42–43
Carbon monoxide, affinity for hemoglobin and myoglobin, 41
Carriers, of thalassemia, 84
Catholic Church, recording of first-
  cousin marriages, 191
Cell, animal, schematic diagram of,
  162
Centrifugal force, nomogram for, 224
Centrifugation, 223–226
 density gradient, 226
 in preparation of globin, 18
 in recovery of red cell membranes, 7
 theoretical aspects of, 223–224
Centrifuge
 in blood sample preparation, 4
 in hemoglobin purification, 14
 in measuring red cell volume, 2
Centromere, 115
Cesium chloride, as gradient in centri-
  fugation, 226
Chance, in genetics. *See* Genetic drift
Chargaff, analysis of DNA, 124
Chemicals, and aplastic anemia, 50
Chiasmata, 117, 118
Child mortality, in first-cousin
  marriages, 195
Chi-square test, 242–244
 and combination of genes, 93
Chloramphenicol
 and aplastic anemia, 50
 as inhibitor of protein synthesis, 172
Chloride shift, and Donnan equi-
  librium, 11

Chromatids, 115
Chromatin
    DNA content of, 144
    use of term, 144
Chromatography, 227–230
    bidimensional, 229
    column, to purify hemoglobin,
        13, 14
    in determining abnormal hemoglobin,
        86
    paper, ascending and descending,
        228
    in purification of proteins, 24
    reverse, 229
    of RNA, and identification of
        nucleotides, 120
    and splitting of hemoglobin
        molecule, 23
    thin-layer, 229
        for amino acid, 18–20
        bidimensional, 20
        in identification of DNP-amino
            acids, 21, 22
Chromosomes
    condensation in mitosis, 115, 116
    human, DNA content of, 144
        after hypotonic treatment, 145
    labeling by ^{3}H-thymidine, 133
        autoradiographs of, 134, 135
    laboratory investigation on,
        141–144
    lengthwise pairing of, in meiosis,
        117
    location of genes, 92, 93
    and locus of nucleolus, 173
    male human, 99
    and Mendel's hypothesis, 117
    potential number of differences, 117
    X, and hereditary conditions, 98
    X and Y, and inheritance of
        anemia, 98
Civilization, and relaxation of
    selection, 194
Cloning, in investigations of sex-linked
    traits, 109
Code(s), of genetic information,
    176–180
    Crick test for, 177–178
Codominance, 80
Codon
    and anticodon, in RNA, 165
    defined, 176

nonsense, 180
Coiling process, of chromosomes
    during mitosis, 144
Coiling-uncoiling process, of chromo-
    somes, 145–147
Colligative properties, of solutions, 6
Color-blindness, 110
Consanguinity
    genetic effects of, 189–190
    taboos and prohibitions against, 191
Continents, and genetic frequencies,
    189
Contingency tables, 245
Cooley's anemia. *See* Thalassemia
Corn, hybrid, as example of maximized
    heterozygosis, 193
Counting chamber, for blood cell
    counts, 3
Counting kit, for blood cells, 2–3
Cousins, marriage of. *See* Con-
    sanguinity
Crossing-over, 117–118
    in chromosomes, 94
    in gene duplication, 96, 97
    homologous and nonhomologous,
        97
Cyclohexamide, as inhibitor of pro-
    tein synthesis, 172
Cytochrome oxidase, affinity for
    oxygen, 40
Cytological map, compared with
    genetic map, 118
Cytosine, structure of, 120, 127

DDT, and control of malaria, 194
DNA. *See* Deoxyribonucleic acid
DNAse action, on DNA, measure-
    ment of, 139–140
DNFB. *See* Dinitrofluorobenzene
DNP-arginine, 21
DNP derivatives, and amino acids, 21
DNP-glycine, 21
DNP-lysine, 21
DNP-protein
    hydrolysis of, 21–22
    preparation of, 21
DPG. *See* Diphosphoglyceric acid
Danielli-Dawson model, for mem-
    brane structure, 7, 8
Deaf-mutism, 195
Death, genetic, 192
    reestablishing equilibrium, 195

Degradation, in establishing
    structure of nucleic acids, 120
Delta chain, of hemoglobin
    molecule, 30
Denaturation, and changes in
    molecular structure, 35–36
Deoxyribonucleic acid, 119, 120
  biosynthesis of, 148
  chemical formula for, 128, 129
  and chromosomes, 144–152
  complete synthesis of, 178–179
  Feulgen's method of detection of,
    120
  homology in different mammals,
    162
  influence of preparations on in-
    corporation of nucleotides, 156
  molecular weight formula, 139
  "nicked," repair by polymerase,
    150
  preparation for study of properties,
    137
  properties of, laboratory investiga-
    tion, 135–140
  ratios of purines to pyrimidines,
    127
  and self-duplication of genetic
    materials, 128
  structure and replication, 140–141
  structure of, genetic implications
    of, 128–132
  techniques for study of distribution
    of, 123–124
  Watson-Crick model, 124–132, 136
Deoxyribonucleic acid polymerase,
    147–152
  in DNA replication, 151
  products of synthesis, 150
Deoxyribonucleic acid-ribonucleic
    acid molecule, hybrid, 160
2-Deoxyribose, 119
Diamond code, of Gamow, 176
Digits, extra, and Older Order of
    Amish, 189
Dinitrofluorobenzene, reaction with
    amino acids, 21, 24
Dinitrophenol. *See* DNP
Diphosphoglyceric acid, and oxyhemo-
    globin dissociation curve, 40–41
Dissociation, of protein molecules, 219
Distribution curves, for heads and
    tails probabilities, 240

Dominance, phenomenon of, 79–80
Dominant traits, 77–78, 79–80
Donnan equilibrium, 9–11
Drying, process in hemoglobin de-
    termination, 13
DuPraw, model for chromosome ul-
    trastructure, 145, 146
DuVigneau, and molecular structure
    of oxytocin, 26
Dwarfism
  chondrodystrophic, 192
  and Older Order of Amish, 189

East Africa, incidence of sickle-cell
    trait in, 204
Ectodermal dysplasia, 110
Egyptian dynasties, inbreeding of,
    191
Electric potential, and Donnan equi-
    librium, 10, 11
Electrode
  glass, 232–233
  standard, in pH determination, 233
Electron microscope
  in determining molecular weight, 22
  technique for examining fine struc-
    tures, 7, 9
Electrophoresis, 219–222
  in determining abnormal hemo-
    globin, 86
  disc, 221–222
  free, 219–221
  paper, 221
  and hemoglobin tests, 53
Embryo, hemoglobin in, 85. *See also*
    Hemoglobin, fetal
Endonuclease, and "nicked" DNA, 151
Endoplasmic reticulum, 161, 163
Entropoietin, 49
Environment
  control of, effect on genetic adap-
    tation, 189
  and understanding of selection, 198
Enzyme(s)
  activation of amino acids for pro-
    tein synthesis, 163
  digestive, in identification of pep-
    tides, 26
  in DNA replication, 147, 150
  enzyme 5.4, 163
  in linking of small DNA strands, 151
  phospholipase C, 7

in protein synthesis, 171
in RNA synthesis, 153–154
in study of DNA and RNA, 120,
    123–124
transcribing DNA from RNA
    template, 181
ultraviolet repair, 152
Epsilon chains, of hemoglobin, 85
Equilibrium
    approach to, and molecular
        weight, 225
    genetic, and Hardy-Weinberg law,
        186
    population in, proportion of
        genotypes in, 187
    reestablished by selection, 195
    sedimentation, in determining
        molecular weight, 225
Erdman's method (reagent), for amino
    acid sequencing, 26, 27
Erythropoiesis, increased, in
    hereditary spherocytosis, 59
Erythropoietin, 49
    and hemoglobin synthesis, 180–182
Eugeny, 196–197
    negative, 196
    positive, 197
Euthanasia, and negative eugeny, 196
Evolutionary tree, and hemoglobin
    chains, 30
Exchange diffusion, 12

Females, vs. males, and transmission
    of hemolytic anemia, 97–100
Ferritin, 51
Ferrous sulphate, to correct iron
    deficiency, 51
Fertility decrease, effects of
    dominant and recessive genes,
    192–193
Fetus, hemoglobin of. *See* Hemo-
    globin, fetal
Fisher, Emil, and structure of
    proteins, 24
Folded-fiber model, for chromosome
    ultrastructure, 145, 146
Folic acid, deficiency of, and
    anemia, 52
Formyl-methionyl-tRNA, and
    protein synthesis, 169
Fraser, model for nucleic acid
    structure, 125

Freezing point, of solutions, 6

G.-6-P. D. *See* Glucose-6-phosphate-
    dehydrogenase
Gamma chain, of hemoglobin
    molecule, 30, 85–86
    and infant death by asphyxia, 54
Garrod, lecture on metabolic
    defects, 152
Gas law, and osmotic pressure
    formula, 6
Gel filtration, as mechanism in
    chromatography, 230
Gene frequency, calculation of,
    186–187
Genes, 77
    deleterious, in first-cousin
        marriages, 195
    lethal. *See* Lethon
    linked, 93
        genetic distance of, 118
    ratios of, 81–83
    recombinations of, frequency of,
        118
    segregation by assortment of
        chromosomes, 93
Genetic counseling, 84–85
    data for, 196
    group discussion on, 100
Genetic drift, 189
Genetic information, 114
    chemical composition of, 118–124
    two ways of storing, 123
Genetic load, 195–196
Genetic map, construction of, 118
Genetic pool, of man, control of,
    by man, 197
Genetics
    human, hypothetical experiment,
        186
    laboratory investigation, 83–84
    population. *See* Population genetics
Genotype(s), 78
    in population in equilibrium, effect
        of consanguinity, 192
    prediction of, 187
    proportion of, effect of increased
        fitness of heterozygote, 193
Geographic location, and sickle-cell
    trait, 199, 200
Ghosts, 7
Glass, pH-sensitive, 232

Globin
    defects in, 53—55
    preparation of, 18
Glucose
    mediated transport for, 11—12
    in preservation of red blood cells,
        55
Glucose-6-phosphate-dehydrogenase
        activity, microdeterminations
        of, 104
Glucose-6-phosphate-dehydrogenase
        deficiency, 102—110
Gortner and Grendel, and recovery of
        red cell membranes, 7
Gower's hemoglobin, 180
Glycerin
    hypertonic, and hemolysis of red
        cells, 6
    to prevent ice crystal formation, 13
Glycine, and related compounds, 38
Greece
    frequency of sickle-cell trait, 199,
        200
    incidence of thalassemia, 205
Growth hormone, and Merrifield's
        method, 31
Guanine
    pairing with cystosine, 131
    structure of, 120, 127

Haploid cells, 117
Hardy-Weinberg Law, 186—189
    methods of testing, 188
Hayden solution, in counting blood
        cells, 2
Hematin, isolated from hemoglobin,
        23
Heme
    amino acid pocket, surrounded by,
        36
    bond structure of, 41
    formation of, 51
    molecular structure of, 23
Hemocytometer, 3
Hemoglobin(s)
    A, 30, 47, 86
    A, S, A$_2$ and B$_2$, recombination
        by crossing-over, 96
    A$_2$, 30, 47, 86
        in thalassemia, 54
    abnormal
        determination of, 86—91

examples of, 86—87
    genetic control in, 91—92
alkaline resistance of, test for, 53
as buffer, 18
    in carbon dioxide transport, 43
C, gene frequency of, and malaria,
        194
constant spring, 180
content of red cells, laboratory
        investigation, 13—15
F, 47
fetal, 30, 85—86
    in adult, 91—92
    affinity for oxygen, 40
    and resistance to malaria, 205
    synthesis, 181
    in thalassemia, 54
Gower I, 85
    as fetal hemoglobin, 30
Gower II, 85
H, 54
inheritance of, 87—91
iron requirements for, 50
molecular structure of, 22—38
molecular weight of, 22—23
normal values for, 14
oxidation, in studies of G.-6-P.D.-
        deficient cells, 103
and permeability of red cell
        membrane, 6
physiological role of, 39—43
primary structure of chains, 28
properties of, laboratory investiga-
        tion of, 38
purification process, 13
relationship to disease, 47—73
S, 82
    and alpha-thalassemia family
        pedigree, 91
    and beta-thalassemia family
        pedigree, 90
    gene frequency of, and malaria,
        194
S and B$_2$, family pedigrees, 92,
        94, 95
S and C, family pedigree, 87
S and E, family pedigree, 88
S, C, and Memphis, family pedigree,
        91
sickle-cell, and malaria parasite,
        204
    in sickle-cell anemia, 79, 80, 198

solubility of, test for, 53
structure of, laboratory investigation, 18—22
structure and properties of, 17
synthesis of, 180—183
genetic control of, 85—87
Hemoglobin chains. *See also* Alpha
chains; Beta chains; *etc.*
abnormalities of, 86
in determining abnormal hemoglobin, 86
evolution by gene duplication,
96, 97
five types of, 85, 86
four chains of, spatial position
of, 37
Hemoglobin lepore, 96
Hemoglobinuria, paroxysmal nocturnal, 56
Hemolysis
defined, 6
prevention of, in freezing of red
cells, 13
Hemolysis-inducing drug, and experimental anemia, 49
Hemophilia, 98—100
carriers of, 98
Hemosiderin, 51
Henderson-Hasselbach equation, 236
Heparin, use in taking blood sample,
2
Hereditary traits
laboratory investigation, 78
ratios of, 81—83
Heterozygosis
chances in first-cousin marriages,
191
increasing, factors in, 197
percentage of, 195
Heterozygotes, 77
distinguished from homozygotes,
82
double, for G.-6-P. D. deficiency and
sickle-cell trait, 109
increase of fitness of, 193
and malaria, 194
Histogram, of probability distribution, 240
Histones, 122—123
discovery of, 119
Homogeneity test, 244—245

Homozygosis
in first-cousin marriages, 192, 195
vs. heterozygosis, and sickle-cell
gene, 198—199
Homozygotes, and malaria, 194
Hormone activity, structure requirements for, 26
Horse, compared to man, myoglobin
and hemoglobin primary structure, 28—29
Huxley, Julian, and positive eugeny,
197
Hybridization, of DNA and RNA,
160—161
Hybrids. *See* Heterozygotes
Hydrochloric acid
and reduction of iron in stomach, 50
titration of, 233—234
Hydrogen bonds
in alpha helix, 33
of DNA chains, 129
between water molecules, 31
Hydrogen ion, in dissociation of
water, 231
Hydrolysis, in determining abnormal
hemoglobin, 86

Ice, hydrogen bonds in, 31
Imferon, in studies of red blood cell
fragility, 65
Inbreeding, reasons for decrease in,
191
Inbreeding coefficient, 190
India, percent of first-cousin marriages,
191
Indian aboriginal groups, frequency
of sickle-cell trait, 199
Infertility, caused by dominant gene,
192
Ingram, and sickle cell anemia, 54
Insulin
molecular structure of, Sanger's
work, 24, 26
synthetic, 30
Ion exchange, as mechanism in chromatography, 230
Ion exchange resins, 230
Iron
absorption of, 50
combining with oxygen, 39
deficiency

Iron, deficiency – *(Continued)*
  causes of, 51
  as public health problem, 51
  from destroyed red blood cells, 50
  electronic configuration of atoms,
    in hemoglobin and oxyhemo-
    globin, 41, 42
  in hematin, 23
  in hemoglobin, 13, 17
    percentage, 22, 23
  metabolism of, 47
  normal content for adult man, 50
  parenteral, in iron deficiency, 51
  procedure for determination of
    content, 14
  toxicity of, 51
  utilization of Fe^{59} for red cell
    formation, 63, 66, 71–72
Isolation, and differences in gene
  frequencies, 189
Isopynic density gradient centrifugation, 226
Isotonic concentrations, and red
  blood cells, 6
Italy
  and sickle-cell trait, 200
  and thalassemia, 205

Japan, percent of first-cousin
  marriages, 191

KOCN. *See* Potassium cyanate
Kidneys, and production of ery-
  thropoietin, 49
Kossel, discovery of histones, 119

Laboratory investigations
  blood and bone marrow smears,
    56–57
  on chromosomes, 141–144
  diagnosis of anemia, 52–53
  experimental anemia, 48
  hemoglobin content of red cells,
    13–15
  of hereditary traits, 78
  human genetics, 83–84
  properties of DNA, 135–140
  properties of hemoglobin, 38
  of red blood cells, 2–5
  on structure of hemoglobin,
    18–22
Lampbrush chromosomes, 173, 175

Lead poisoning, and biosynthesis
  of protoporphyrin, 51
Least squares, method of, 246
Lethon, 196
Leukocyte counts, in sickle-cell-
  malaria experiments, 202, 203
Ligases. *See* Selases
Linear relationships, of data, 245–246
Lipids, and permeability of substances,
  7
Lipoprotein membrane, 7–9

Malaria
  association with hemoglobin defects,
    193–194
  and sickle-cell trait, 200
Man, as population in equilibrium,
  189
Manometer, for osmotic pressure.
  See Osmometer
Marriage, first-cousin. *See* Consanguinity
Mating, random, and genetic calculations, 188
Mean, calculation of, 241
Medical history, questionnaire on,
  211–217
Megaloblastic anemia. *See* Anemia,
  pernicious
Meiosis, 115–116
  pairing of chromosomes in, and
    segregation of genes, 117
  schematic representation of, 116
Membrane(s)
  properties of, 7
  recovered by centrifugation. *See*
    Ghosts
  red blood cell, defects in, and
    anemia, 55–56
  structure of, 5–9
  tests of fragility of, 56
Mendel's laws, and hereditary diseases,
  77–78
Merrifield's method, for polypeptide
  synthesis, 30–31
Meselson-Stahl experiment, 141–143
Messenger RNA, 153
Metabolic defects
  and anemia, 55
  in hereditary spherocytosis, 71
Metals, heavy, molecular study of, 32
Methemoglobin, 55

microdeterminations of, 104
reduction of
  by red blood cells to hemo-
    globin, 55
  experiments, 104–106
Methemoglobinemia, 55
Methylamine, 38
Methylene blue solution, in staining
  blood cells, 4
3-0-methyl-glucose, as by-product in
  glucose transport, 12
Micropipette, in counting blood
  cells, 2–3
Microscope. *See also* Electron
  microscope
  for blood cell counts, 3–4
Microspectrophotometers, in study
  of DNA and RNA, 124
Microspectrophotometric methods,
  for study of intracellular
  structure, 144
Miescher, work with cell nuclei,
  118–119
Migration
  electrophoretic, of large molecules,
    220
  of samples, in chromatography, 229
Migratory movements, and random
  marriage, 189
Millipore-filtration studies, of sickle
  cells, 103
Mitochondria, resemblance to
  bacteria, 172
Mitosis, 114–115
  schematic representation of, 115
Molecular diameter, and permeability
  of red cell membrane, 6–7
Molecular weight
  determination of, 22
    by centrifugation, 224–225
  of macromolecules, determined by
    acrylamine electrophoresis, 222
Molecules
  dissociation by electrophoresis,
    219–222
  intrinsic viscosity, 139
  migration through membranes, 7, 10
Mosaic model, of Braton and Singer,
  for membrane structure, 9
Mosaicism, 110
Muller, and positive eugeny, 197
Mutation, 194–195

and natural selection, 198
rate of, 195
  estimation of, 195
  and replacement of sickle-cell
    genes, 199
  spontaneous, in Watson-Crick
    model, 132
Mutational load, 195
Myoglobin, 27
  affinity for oxygen, 39–40
  primary structure of chains, 28
  tridimensional structure of, 34, 35

Nearest-neighbor analysis, of Kornberg,
  148, 149
Neurospora, study of mutants of, 153
Newborn
  hemoglobin of, 30
  and resistance to malaria, 205
Ninhydrin, as reagent for amino
  acids, 20
Nitrogen bases, common to tRNA, 165
Nucleic acid(s)
  purines and pyrimidines in, 120
  structure of, 122
    discovery of primary, 163
  studies of, 119
Nucleolar organizer, 173
Nucleolus
  base composition of, 173
  mutant strains lacking, 173–174
Nucleotide(s)
  in biosynthesis of DNA, 148
  in RNA, 120, 121
  structure of, 121, 129
    secondary, 163, 164
Nucleus, as storage place of genetic
  information, 120
Null hypothesis, 242
Nutritional deficiencies, and anemia, 52

Ochoa's enzyme, 153–154
Osmometer, 5
Osmosis, defined, 5
Osmotic imbalance, in Donnan
  equilibrium, 10
Osmotic pressure, of solutions, 5–6
Overton, discovery of red cell
  permeability, 6–7
Oxygen
  affinity curve, myoglobin vs.
    hemoglobin, 40

Oxygen–*(Continued)*
  volume used by man, 39
Oxygen transport, 17
  by hemoglobin, 39
Oxyhemoglobin dissociation curve,
  shifts in, 40, 41
Oxytocin, molecular structure of, 26

pH
  of blood, and paroxysmal nocturnal
    hemoglobinuria, 56
  change during titration, 234
  determination of, 232–233
  and dissociation of proteins, 219
pH meter, 233
PTC. *See* Phenyl thicarbamide
Partition, as mechanism in chroma-
    tography, 229
Pascal triangle, 237–239
Pauling
  interest in nucleic acids, 125
  and sickle-cell anemia, 54, 153
Pauling and Corey, and structure of
    nucleic acid, 125
Peas, crossing of, and Mendel's laws,
    77–78
Pedigrees, family
  in determining abnormal hemo-
    globin, 86–91
  model for, 79
  in sickle-cell anemia, 79, 80
Penicillin, and aplastic anemia, 50
Peptide bond(s), 32
  formation of, 26
  linking amino acids, 17, 24
Peptidyl-puromycin, formation of, 172
Permeability
  of red cell membranes, 5, 6–7,
    10, 11
  mediated transport, 11–12
Permease
  defined, 11
  for glucose, 11, 12
  for glycerin, 12, 13
Pernicious anemia. *See under*
    Anemia(s)
Phagocytic cells, in red blood cell
    destruction, 49
Phenotype, 78
Phenyl thicarbamide
  capability of tasting, in genetic
    experiment, 186, 188

  as hereditary trait, 78, 81
  taste-blindness gene, frequency of,
    189, 190
Phenylbutazone, and aplastic anemia,
    50
Phenylhydrazine, in experimental
    anemia, 48
Phenylisothiocyanate, in amino acid
    sequencing, 26, 27
Phenylthiohidantoin, in amino acid
    sequencing, 27
Phloridzin, as inhibitor of sugar up-
    take, 11, 12
Photocolorimetric method, of hemo-
    globin determination, 13
Phospholipase C, and digestion of
    membranes, 7
Phospholipid molecules, polar and
    nonpolar ends, 7, 8
Phosphorus, radioactive, in study of
    genetic information storage, 123
Plasma bicarbonate, carbon dioxide
    transported as, 42
Plasmodium falciparum, and sickle-
    cell trait, 201, 202, 206
Pneumococcus, experiments with R
    and S strain, 124
Polar groups, in hemoglobin and myo-
    globin molecules, 35
Polyglycine, 33
Polymorphism, balanced, 195
Polynucleotide precursors, 131, 132
Population genetics, 185–206
Potassium
  concentration, and red blood cells, 5
  in plasma, 9–11
  in red cells, 9–11
Potassium chloride, in pH determina-
    tion, 233
Potassium cyanate, and reversal of
    sickling, 85
Pregnancy, iron needs in, 50
Primaquine, and susceptibility to
    hemolytic anemia, 97
Primer, role in DNA replication, 147,
    148
Probabilities, 237–246
Proline, structure of, 34
Protamines, 122–123
  isolation by Miescher, 119
Protein
  amino acids in, 24, 25

as building blocks of body, 114
defined, 17
dissociation by electrophoresis,
219–222
hydrolysis, 18
molecules, 7
for production of red blood cells, 49
relationship to genetic information,
152
and storage of genetic information,
123
in storage of iron, 51
in transportation of iron, 50
tridimensional structure of, 17
ultracentrifugation process, 22
Protein synthesis
amino acid sequence, 27
Dintzis model for, 165, 166, 167
inhibitors of, 172
schematic representation of, 171
Protoporphyrin, in formation of
heme, 51
Purines
and pyrimidines, pairing in DNA
chains, 129, 130
structure of, 119, 120, 127
Puromycin
and amino acid tRNA, structural
similarity, 172
as inhibitor of protein synthesis,
172
Pyknotic stage, of red blood cell, 48
Pyrimidines, structure of, 119, 120,
127

RNA. *See* Ribonucleic acid
mRNA. *See* Messenger RNA
tRNA. *See* Transfer RNA
Race, and differences in gene frequencies, 189
Radiation, ionizing, and aplastic
anemia, 50
Recessive disease, surveys of, 83
Recessive traits, 78
Red blood cells
abnormalities of
laboratory tests for, 52
role in hereditary spherocytosis,
70–73
carbon dioxide transport, 42
chromium-labeled, osmotic and
mechanical fragility of, 66–70

counting of, 2–3
deficiency in production of, as cause
of anemia, 49
destruction process, 48–49
enzyme-deficient, 102, 109
Fe59-labeled
mechanical fragility of, 65
osmotic fragility of, 64
hemoglobin content of, 23
increased destruction of, as cause of
anemia, 49
investigation of hemoglobin content,
13–15
laboratory investigation of, 2–5
measuring volume of, 2
mechanical fragility, method of determining, 60, 63
membrane structure, 5–9
normal values for, 4
number of in body, 49
osmotic fragility
in hereditary spherocytosis, 59–73
test for, 52
permeability of, 5–6
preservation of, 13
production of, 48
relationship to disease, 47–73
staining for examination, 4
Regression, 246
Religions, and consanguinity, 191
Renaturation, of protein molecular
structure, 36
Reticulocyte, 48
Retinoblastoma, frequency of, 194
Reverse transcriptase, 181
Rhodesia, Northern, malaria and
sickle-cell trait in, 200
Ribonucleic acid, 119
alkaline hydrolysis of, 121
alkaline transfer reaction with, 155
distribution of, techniques for study
of, 123–124
as primer for DNA replication, 152
soluble, role of, 161–165
Ribonucleotides, enzymatic incorporation into RNA, 154–159
Ribose, 119
Ribosomes, 151
and nucleolus, 173–176
number per cell, 173
and protein synthesis, 165–173
in red blood cell formation, 48

Ribosomes—*(Continued)*
  reticulocyte, electron micrographs of, 170
Rifomycin, in study of RNA, 160
Robertson, work with membrane layers, 7
Rotors, designs of, for centrifugation, 225

Sanger, and splitting of hemoglobin molecule, 24
Saturation curves, hemoglobin, myoglobin and cytoglobin, 39
Sedimentation coefficient, determination of, 224, 226
Sedimentation rate, 223
  in determining molecular weight, 22
Segregational load, 195—196
Selases, in linking of small DNA strands, 151
Selection
  effect on dominant and recessive traits, 193
  effect on equilibrium, 192—195
  and estimation of mutations, 195
  and spread of genes in population, 198
Selection pattern, and malaria, 194
Selective advantage, and sickle-cell trait, 199—200
Self-duplication, of genetic material, mechanism for, 128, 131
Self-evaluation tests
  anemia, 57—58
  answers to, 247—249
  genetics and anemia, 100—101
  on genetic information storage, 182—183
  molecular structure of hemoglobin, 43—44
  on population genetics, 197
  red cell investigation, 15
Sephadex, in determining molecular weight, 22
Sephadex G-25, in hemoglobin purification, 13
Serebrovsky, and positive eugeny, 197
Sex determination, and chromosomes, 117
Sex-linked genes, inactivation of loci, 109
Sex-linked traits, 97—100

Sickle-cell trait. *See also* Anemia, sickle-cell
  distinguishing between carriers and patients, 198
  protection against malaria, 198—200
Sickling, of red blood cells, 54, 79
Sigma factor, 160
Silica gel, in thin-layer chromatography, 19
Sister exchange, between chromosomes, 135, 136
Smears
  blood, laboratory investigation of, 56—57
  bone marrow, laboratory investigation of, 56
Sodium
  in plasma, 9—11
  in red cells, 9—11
Sodium chloride
  in blood sample preparation, 4
  isotonic concentration, and red blood cells, 6
Solutions
  boiling point elevation, 6
  freezing point depression, 6
  osmotic pressure of, 5—6
Species, of man, and variety of gene frequencies, 189
Spectrophotometer, in microdeterminations, 104
Spectrum, absorption, of hemoglobin, 38
Spherocytosis, 48
  hereditary, 55—56, 59—73, 206
    distribution of Fe[59] in, 63
    presplenectomy studies, 61—66
    splenectomy and post-splenectom studies, 66—70
Spleen
  enlarged
    in hereditary spherocytosis, 71
    and sickle-cell trait, 200
  in hereditary spherocytosis, 70—73
  in red blood cell destruction, 48—49
  removal of
    for correction of hemolytic process, 66
    in hereditary spherocytosis, 59
    and red blood cell defects, 56
  as source of fragile red blood cells, 73

Spleen-drip cells
  postsplenectomy survival of, 70
  studies of osmotic and mechanical
    fragility, 66–70
Splenectomy. *See* Spleen, removal of
Splenic sinuses, 49
Splenomegaly. *See* Spleen, enlarged
Stain, for red blood cell examina-
    tion, 4
Standard deviation, formula for, 241
Standard error, 242
Statistics, 237–246
Sterilization, compulsory, and nega-
    tive eugeny, 196
Straight line, in data relationships,
    245–246
Study guides
  on anemia, 47
  genetic information, 113–114
  Mendel's laws and genetics, 77
  population genetics, 185
  red cell investigation, 1
  structure and properties of hemo-
    globin, 17–18
Sucrose
  as gradient in centrifugation, 226
  isotonic concentration, and red
    blood cells, 6
  and permeability of red cell mem-
    brane, 6
Sugars, and penetration of red cells,
    11, 12
Sulfonilamide, and susceptibility to
    hemolytic anemia, 97
Sutton, and parallel of genes and
    chromosomes, 117
Svedberg equation, for sedimentation
    coefficient, 224

t Test, 242, 243
TLC. *See* Chromatography, thin-layer
Target cells, in thalassemia, 53
Taste blindness. *See also* Phenyl
    thicarbamide
  in genetic experiment, 186, 188
Taylor, experiment with lily root
    tips, 134–135
Temperature
  constant, in chromatography,
    228–229
  and pH meters, 233
Templates

role in DNA replication, 147, 148
  in self-duplication process, 131
Tetracyclines, and aplastic anemia, 50
Thalassemia, 53–54
  beta, abnormal hemoglobin in, 86
  expectancy of, 84, 85
  gene frequency and Hardy-Weinberg
    law, 188–189
  and genetic counseling, 84
  hereditary traits in, 80
Thalassemia gene, and resistance to
    malaria, 205
Thymidine, and ultraviolet damage
    to DNA, 152
Thymine, structure of, 120, 127
Thymonucleic acid, 119
Thymus gland, nucleic acid from.
    See Thymonucleic acid
Thyroid deficiency, and PTC taste-
    blindness, 194
Tiselius apparatus for free electro-
    phoresis, 219, 220
Titration
  of strong acid, 233–234
  of weak acid, 234–235
Triplets, in genetic coding, 176, 177,
    178
Transfer RNA, 165
Transferrin, 50
Transportation, invention of, effect
    on mating population, 189
Trimethadone, and aplastic anemia, 50

Uganda, frequency of sickle-cell trait,
    199, 200
Ultracentrifugation
  in determination of molecular
    weight, 22
  in purification of proteins, 24
  use in studying DNA structure,
    140–141
Ultraviolet absorption
  nomogram for calculating nucleic
    acid and protein concentration
    in solution, 138
  and properties of DNA, 135, 137–138,
    142
Ultraviolet light, in chromatography,
    228
Ultraviolet radiation, damage to
    DNA, 152
Uracil, structure of, 120

Urea
  and hemolysis of red cells, 6
  and splitting of hemoglobin
    molecule, 23

van der Waals forces, in protein
    molecule, 35
Van't Hoff, and osmotic pressure, 5
Variability, importance in evolution
    of species, 197
Vein, procedure for removing blood, 4
Vicia faba, pollen of, and suscep-
    tibility to hemolytic anemia, 97
Viscosimeter, 138–139
Viscosity
  intrinsic, 139
  measurement of, 138–139
Vitamin B_{12}, deficiency of, and
    anemia, 52
von Beneden, Edouard, and meiosis,
    116

Water
  ionization of, 231–232
  molecule, 31

Watson-Crick Model, of molecular
    structure of nucleic acids,
    124–132
Weight, molecular. *See* Molecular
    weight
Wilkins
  and nucleic acids, 125
  x-ray diffraction studies of DNA,
    134
"Wobble" hypothesis, of Crick, 179
Women, iron requirements of, 50

Xeroderma pigmentosum, and lack of
    DNA repair enzyme, 152
X-ray diffraction
  in study of peptide bonds, 32
  and transformation of hemoglobin
    to oxyhemoglobin, 41
D-Xylose, and penetration of red
    cells, 11
L-Xylose, and penetration of red
    cells, 11

Zonal density gradient centrifuga-
    tion, 226